Jacki Winter has been an insulin-dependent diabetic since the age of twenty. Until that time she worked in marketing, but when her illness was diagnosed she gave up her demanding job, and it was then that she discovered the benefits to herself of exercise through keep-fit classes. From these she progressed to teaching what she considers to be the better, gradual way of get fit. She is now a successful teacher of twelve classes a week, attended by a number of diabetics. She and her husband enjoy exercise as relaxation too, especially walking and dancing.

Dr Barbara Boucher is a Consultant Physician at the London Hospital and since 1970 has been running a diabetic clinic there. She also works in a Metabolic Unit, both researching into diabetes and running a service for diabetics. She has published numerous articles on her research in journals such as the *Lancet* and *Diabetologia*. She is married and has two grown-up children. Walking and riding are her favourite forms of exercise.

THE DIABETICS' GET FIT BOOK

Jacki Winter

Introduction by Dr Barbara Boucher
Consultant Physician, the London Hospital

Forewords by Dr Arnold Bloom, MD, FRCP
The British Diabetic Association's Executive
Chairman
and
Sir Harry Secombe, CBE
President of the British Diabetic Association

MARTIN DUNITZ

For all their love, support,
understanding and guidance, I would
like to dedicate this book to my
parents and to my dear husband,
Peter.

J.W.

© Jacki Winter, 1984
© Introduction Barbara Boucher 1984

First published in the United Kingdom in 1984
by Martin Dunitz Limited, London

British Library Cataloguing in Publication Data
Winter, Jacki
    The diabetics' get fit book.
    1. Physical fitness
    I. Title
    613.7   RA781

    ISBN 0–906348–66–8
    ISBN 0–906348–65–X Pbk

Phototypeset in Garamond by Input Typesetting Ltd, London
Printed in Singapore by Toppan Printing Company (S) Pte Ltd

CONTENTS

Keeping fit is important for everybody but particularly so for those
with diabetes. Jacki Winter has diabetes herself and runs keep-fit classes.
She has an easy style and her book is
a little masterpiece of good sense,
sound advice and encouragement for
diabetics of all ages.

Arnold Bloom, MD, FRCP
The British Diabetic Association's
Executive Chairman

When I found out that I was a diabetic I wasn't sure what it was. It was as obscure to me as leprosy and at first I panicked a bit. Then my doctor patiently explained that it was a pretty common disease and that if I was sensible and came down from the roof I could lead a normal life. And so I gradually realized that by dieting and taking exercise, diabetes can be easily controlled. I set about losing weight, and now that I can see my feet again when I'm in a standing position, it's much less difficult to touch them. Playing golf has become an essential part of my weekly curriculum and I walk far more than I have ever done. To be honest, I really believe that in some ways finding out that I was a diabetic was one of the best things that could have happened to me. I have been forced to take care of myself and am fitter now than I have been for many years.

Among the exercises in this book I am particularly interested in the ones involving the legs. There's an old adage in show business that a comic needs good legs – presumably because we need to run faster than our audiences. But *all* the exercises in this book will be a tremendous help to diabetics whether NIDDS or IDDS, and I, for one, will keep plugging away at the Donkey Kick and the Bouncer. Who knows, I may find a new career in ballet?

Sir Harry Secombe, CBE
President, the British Diabetic Association

INTRODUCTION: HOW EXERCISE CAN HELP DIABETES

Diabetes is a common disorder affecting up to 6 per cent of the population in some countries in the Western world. In the United Kingdom there are probably one million and in the USA about 5 million people with it. Diabetes isn't often curable, but when reasonable care is taken to control it, the diabetic usually leads a pretty normal life.

For most diabetics a balance between the energy provided by the food they eat and the energy they use up in daily activities can be achieved by adjusting their diet; for many, however, tablets or insulin injections have to be used as well. As diabetics of course know, it is keeping the balance between these three aspects: the food you eat, your treatment and activity, that is the key to achieving freedom from day-to-day problems and upsets, rather as a three-legged stool can only stand steady when the legs are of equal length. This balance is also useful in reducing risks of long-term complications.

Much has been learnt in recent years about helpful ways to use insulin and tablet treatments in keeping better control, and also about the values of eating more natural carbohydrates and high-fibre foods than used to be thought wise for diabetics. Other books in this series reflect these developments (*Diabetes* by Dr Jim Anderson; *The Diabetics' Diet Book* and the *Diabetics' Cookbook* by Dr Jim Mann and the Oxford team).

This book is concerned with the third 'leg of the stool', that is, with ways that diabetics can build up their exercise. In the past few years the value of returning from our increasingly sedentary Western way of life to more physical activity has been convincingly shown to help reduce the risks of heart and blood vessel diseases. It has also been found that exercise taken regularly and for pleasure is more beneficial than exercise required in your work. Diabetes is linked to these risks so that those with the condition should perhaps be encouraged to join the trend back towards the sort of activity that was usual until the introduction of the car and the television.

Care has to be taken when anyone 'out of training' gets back into exercising, and especially by people with diabetes, because extra exercise changes their balance. Thought has to be given to adjusting to a new balance. Food intake needs to be altered, or if medical treatment is used, that may need changing *before* any new programme of physical exercise is begun. You will want to consult your usual medical adviser to discuss how you will maintain balance and avoid upsetting the diabetes if exercising is new to you. Each chapter in this book includes reminders and practical ways of taking care not to upset your diabetes.

You will have to be clear about how extra exercise can affect your diabetes. Since this will depend mainly on the type of diabetes you have and the treatment you are on, this introductory section tells you about the two main types of diabetes and the problems of balance in each sort. For those with complications, or with other health problems, exercise may need to be approached cautiously. I explain this too, so that you will know what points to raise with your doctor when considering taking up any new form of exercise.

What is diabetes?
Diabetes mellitus means the passing of sweet water and this happens in diabetics because the blood sugar level is higher than usual and this sugar spills over into the urine as blood goes through the kidneys. Blood sugar (glucose) is usually kept down to normal by the hormonal 'messenger' in the blood, insulin. This hormone, made in the pancreas, stops us producing more glucose than we need and ensures that any extra sugars available after eating are directed into body stores, mostly in the liver and muscles, and as fat. Lack of insulin allows sugar (glucose) levels to rise in the bloodstream and be wasted by being lost in the urine.

Insulin-dependent and non insulin-dependent diabetes
Failure of the pancreas to make enough insulin leads to diabetes. This happens quite quickly, often in weeks, perhaps after a virus infection or other injury has damaged the insulin-making cells. Without insulin, diabetics of this sort soon become very unwell, which is why they are described as insulin-dependent. Other, often older people, and those who tend to be overweight, develop diabetes more gradually. They make insulin but it doesn't seem to work as effectively as it should. Diabetics of this sort are called non insulin-dependent since a combination of correct eating and losing any excess weight will improve the diabetes, probably by allowing their insulin to work better. Only with a severe illness is insulin treatment likely to be needed for these diabetics. Insulin production may flag sooner or later in people with this type of diabetes so that they may come to need treatment, either with tablets that increase insulin action, or later with insulin itself.

The blood sugar levels tend to be too high in this type of diabetes if the wrong foods are eaten, excess weight isn't lost or when any usual exercise is missed out. This is also true for insulin-dependent diabetics but they have the added problem of gauging how much insulin they need.

Why keeping control is important
People with both types of diabetes need to keep the glucose, or sugar, in the blood as normal as possible. That is what is usually meant by

9

having the diabetes under control. This correction of blood sugar is important in avoiding complications such as infections and damage to tissues, since it seems that the high blood sugar may itself cause or worsen these problems. The damage that we specially hope to avoid is to the eyes and kidneys, and also to the blood vessels, for example, of the legs and heart.

Exercise for non insulin-dependent diabetics
The way to achieve good balance for most people with this type of diabetes is to eat sensibly and lose any extra weight. Often the older person is less active than before and losing weight becomes more diffi- cult. Regular exercise may make it easier to lose weight, provided any increase in appetite is satisfied with the right foods from the diet plan, and not with unsuitable extras!

Any weight loss produced by more exercise may for diabetics on medication lead to a reduction in the need for tablets. If a diabetic begins exercising regularly and as a result loses weight when on stronger tablets, low blood sugars may occur. Such reactions or 'hypos' are uncommon, but for this reason you should never combine stricter dieting with your new exercises when you are on tablets without consulting your doctor first about possible changes in the tablets.

Increasing exercise can be useful for both non insulin-dependent and insulin-dependent diabetics as it reduces resistance to insulin and this improves the control of blood sugars. Exercise also increases blood flow in the tissues and lowers certain fats in the bloodstream. These effects last long after the exercise itself stops and are a long-term bonus, as in non-diabetics, in reducing the risks of heart and circulatory diseases.

Balance for insulin-dependent diabetics
The diabetic on insulin has a much more difficult balancing act: difficult because meals vary and are digested at different speeds; because insulin has to be given to act over a set length of time and this may vary unexpectedly, and an injection once given can't be taken back. This is a very complicated situation compared to insulin production in non- diabetics which varies all the time to keep the blood glucose steady. Different activities also use energy up at different rates. No wonder that people on insulin often need to readjust their routine, or 'restabilize' and that each person has to adapt his or her routine and treatment individ- ually to achieve a reasonable balance.

Exercise for insulin-dependent diabetics
This has the same benefits in preventing heart and circulatory diseases as it does for non insulin-dependent diabetics and non-diabetics. But for insulin-dependent diabetics the additional problems in taking up exercise are that it uses up sugar while you are active and also afterwards, as your energy stores are rebuilt. If the blood sugar is allowed to fall too low,

reactions or 'hypos' will develop and can be severe. Since this is very undesirable and unpleasant, as anyone on insulin will know, and since it is also an avoidable risk, those of you who are on insulin must be sure you know how hypos can be avoided.

Avoiding hypos while exercising As an insulin-dependent diabetic you can use either of the following plans or a combination of the two. But you must first have the agreement of your usual medical adviser.

1. Consider reducing the amount of insulin on board by giving less in the relevant injection. For example, for those on two daily insulin injections, exercise can be anticipated by taking a smaller dose of insulin before the planned exercise session. For those on insulin pumps the rate of administration could be cut (or even stopped for vigorous exercise). For those on once daily insulin though, cutting the single dose back may not be helpful if it causes the blood sugar to be too high at other times of day.

2. Consider also taking enough extra food before you exercise to cover both the amount of physical work you will do and the recovery period when your sugars continue to be burnt up at a faster rate (see page 18). This method is often used by those on once a day insulin and may be combined with planned cuts in the insulin dose.

   Take care that what you eat is sufficiently nourishing but not too heavy or indigestible, since exercising on a full stomach can stop you absorbing the snack properly.

Long-term effects of exercise
Changing from a sedentary lifestyle to regular vigorous activity will not only alter balance during and shortly after exercise but may reduce the amount of insulin needed each day. Should you come to enjoy regular exercise and find a tendency to reactions at times not related to exercise and without other explanations, then you may need to consider further reduction in each of your insulin injections. Your doctor will be able to help sort this out.

If later you stop exercising, for example, after a sprain, or if you have flu, do not forget that insulin needs may well rise to what they were before.

When should you be careful about exercise?

1. For diabetics on insulin who are not yet in balance, or who may be out of control with quite high blood sugars, exercise may worsen things. Clearly no one with newly diagnosed diabetes or newly on

11

insulin should go into exercise until he or she feels ready for it, and has the doctor's agreement on that point.

2. Any diabetic who is unwell or off-colour should give planned exercise a miss until he or she is better.

3. Those who know they have diabetic complications should avoid vigorous exercise because of the danger of leaky blood vessels, especially if eye problems develop.

4. Insulin-dependent diabetics who have had the condition for ten to fifteen years may have some complications without knowing it and should ask their doctor about this before undertaking new and vigorous exercise.

5. Those with non insulin-dependent diabetes may have had the condition longer than they think and they should also consult their doctor for the same reasons as in 4.

For anyone with these problems, gentler activity such as walking may be better than competitive sports or communal exercise sessions.

Other health problems
People with diabetes can have other health problems. If you are under thirty and have kept pretty active, you can probably increase your activity without risk. Those over thirty who are rather sedentary, who have become overweight, or anyone who is on any sort of medication or surveillance for any chronic medical problem should consult his or her usual medical adviser before taking up any new and vigorous physical exercise. Walking can usually be taken up by anyone, provided it is comfortable.

What exercise to choose?
It is hard to think of any sport or other form of exercise that has not been successfully undertaken by diabetics. There are international footballers on insulin, there have been Wimbledon champions, and many professional sportsmen with diabetes. It is up to you to choose a form of activity that attracts you, that you know you can cope with, and will want to continue. Taking up a suitable keep-fit programme like the one in this book will teach you how to exercise safely and enjoyably. Exercise done as recreation is also far better for your health than any imposed by your work. Provided that neither you nor your doctor find any reason for exercise to be difficult, dangerous or uncomfortable for you, you can work out a programme to suit your tastes, your age and abilities from among the suggestions in the chapters that follow.

DR BARBARA BOUCHER
Consultant Physician, the London Hospital

1   PREPARING TO GET FIT

There is no doubt that living with diabetes is not quite as simple as we may like to believe. The diabetic, whatever his or her age, will occasionally feel low and bored with the continual routine of controlling diet and energy and testing for sugar – but on the positive side, diabetes can be a help. No longer will you take good health for granted and rarely will you abuse your system by bingeing on unnecessary sweets and gâteaux. Probably you will aim much harder for peak physical fitness, as if to counteract the fact that you are living with this condition.

For my own part, diabetes has given me a framework to live in. I have my low days too, but generally I keep positive; I treat my body kindly, appreciate a healthy diet and enjoy the benefits of regular physical exercise.

There is no need to become fanatical about any one aspect, but I hope that having this book near by will help keep you on the positive tracks to a long, fit and enjoyable life.

Now that you've decided to start a get-fit routine, you need to think carefully about where to begin, how much exercise you should do, what type suits you best. In this chapter you'll find practical advice for starting regular exercise, whatever your age and level of fitness.

Personal assessment
Would you say you are fit? How do you assess what being fit actually is? Medically, it is judged by how fast your heartbeat returns to its normal rate after vigorous exercise. This is known as heart recovery rate. But it is also of course related to such factors as your age, sex and general state of health. As a diabetic you may think you are rather 'delicate'. Certainly you have a condition to take care of, but there is no reason why you cannot be as fit as any non-diabetic. As an insulin-dependent diabetic myself, I can honestly say that I am fitter now than I have ever been before. When I was at school I was considered lazy where physical activity and sports were concerned. Yet since the onset of diabetes I have managed to reach a level of fitness where I can spend a few hours each day exercising without strain or upset to my diabetic routine.

You hardly need to do as much exercise as that, but keeping as fit as your age and general condition allows will help you towards a healthy, cheerful state of mind and reduce the chances of complications. There are plenty of different ways to exercise, from the gentle forms such as walking to energetic sports like football and squash. The get-fit workout that forms the main part of this book can be adapted for anyone and you build it up as you increase your fitness level.

Ask yourself the following questions.

1. Are you more than 14 lb (6 kg) overweight (see page 17)?
2. Do you smoke?
3. Have you failed to do any regular physical activity outside your basic routine during the past year?
4. Do you get out of breath if you try to rush upstairs or hurry for a bus?

If you say yes to two or more of these questions, you are not as fit as you could be. If you become breathless by just hurrying upstairs or for a bus, and you are under fifty, it's likely that there is room for improvement! The same applies if when you stand naked in front of a mirror you feel less than satisfied with your shape.

Before you undertake more physical activity remember that your current condition has not come about overnight but may have taken many years to develop, so similarly you should embark on your exercise regime slowly and in planned steps, since fitness too takes time to build up. Don't expect miracles; nevertheless I am sure you will be surprised at how quickly you begin to feel the benefit of exercise.

Do you smoke? If this is one of the questions you answered yes to, let me put in my word, even if you are bored by hearing the advice: you should attempt to cut out smoking completely. There is now a lot of social and medical pressure on people not to smoke; smoking is the cause of 60,000 deaths each year in the UK alone. For diabetics it is even less desirable since it aggravates arterial disease, one of the associated problems of diabetes, and it also increases the risk of diabetic eye damage. It is often said that smoking helps to alleviate stress and tension. Well, exercise does this too, without all the dangers and disadvantages of smoking.

Are you newly diagnosed or poorly stabilized?
One important point to bear in mind for people who have discovered they are diabetic only in the past few weeks: most of the guidelines and exercises in this book are aimed at the diabetic person who is stabilized. Very often, the first month or so of coping with diabetes is difficult and you may find that your stamina is at a low ebb, but fairly quickly your insulin treatment (whether dosage and/or diet) will be sorted out, enabling you to put exercise into your daily life. Remember, if in doubt your diabetic doctor will be glad to reassure you.

It may be that you have been diabetic for some time and that you have recently had problems keeping yourself well stabilized. When your diabetic balance is poor due to illness or a change in lifestyle, vigorous exercise can actually worsen the situation. If you are in the process of restabilization you should check with your doctor on when you are ready to begin a regular exercise regime.

What are the special advantages of exercise for the diabetic?

Circulation
One of the most common problems associated with diabetes is poor circulation, and sometimes reduced sensation goes with it. This can show itself in several ways – the inability to feel the difference between hot and cold, especially in the feet, generalized pain and sometimes a pins-and-needles feeling in the legs, feet or toes. Minor cuts, infections like athlete's foot, and blisters are likely to take more time to heal and in the meantime they may become infected. Septic infections can be dangerous if not professionally treated, as gangrene may result. All foot injuries should be treated as quickly as possible and during treatment maintaining circulation is vitally important (I give more advice on looking after your feet on pages 24–5). Gentle exercise can help, although you should check with your doctor that this is right for you and you are doing the right sort. Exercising both hands and feet helps ward off chilblains, which are a danger as they can lead to infections.

Looking after your hands generally and keeping the circulation going is equally important. Don't forget to wear gloves during the winter and make a point of doing the hand exercises on page 46–7 whenever you think about it.

Relaxation
For a diabetic, learning to relax is essential for maintaining good blood sugar control. Think how disruptive to your sugar balance it can be to lose your temper often and find yourself unable to cope with everyday problems, anxieties or family quarrels.

When you are in this mood your pulse rate increases and your body has to work a lot harder to cope with any alarming or unexpected situation: your heart pounds, your blood pressure is raised so that more blood is pumped to the muscles, heart and brain. Adrenaline is released and sugar comes from the liver to provide fuel for the muscles. You may sweat as your body's cooling system comes into play and there are changes in the electrical resistance in the skin. Imagine the effect this has on your blood sugar level. Your sugars may be lowered more rapidly than normal so that hypos (insulin reactions) can occur. In the diabetic with stresses at work or at home, blood sugars are also likely to become un-stable due to the stress itself and also to irregular eating or perhaps bingeing on the wrong types of food, and once again the long-term health will be at risk. How can you overcome these risks by exercising?

Part of the art of relaxing is through learning to breathe gently and calmly, and the exercises in the cool-down section in Chapter 4 show how you can do this by yourself. Many of the other excercises in this book are extremely beneficial in releasing tension, especially the head, neck, shoulder and arm exercises (see pages 42, 48). They can be done anywhere, at home or in the office, whenever you are feeling very pent up.

Relaxation is a vast topic and is worth a little extra reading. Jane Madders's *Stress and Relaxation*, also in this series, is full of useful hints, information and exercises and is excellent reading for all ages.

Ways to relax

1. Don't try too hard to relax as this may itself make you tense.
2. Don't believe that you have to make your mind blank in order to relax. It's almost impossible to do. Instead, breathe slowly and gently and think of each part of your body, relaxing the muscle groups from toes upwards.
3. Don't think that it is necessary to set aside thirty minutes each day to lie down in a dark room. You can learn to relax just as well during a two-minute period sitting on a chair anywhere.
4. Don't believe that your favourite sport or pastime is relaxation. Playing cards, chess, watching a film or knitting are all activities which may make you feel quite tense.
5. If you have got time to lie down and rest for a few minutes each day, try lying with your feet and legs propped up above your waist level so that the blood drains back to your heart. Support the whole length of your legs not to strain the back of your knees. This is particularly recommended for pregnant women and people who suffer from varicose veins, but anyone will feel immensely relaxed after a few minutes in this position.

Weight

A lot of diabetics, particularly the non insulin-dependent, are overweight and are advised by their doctors to reduce gradually and sensibly. If you have been told to lose a few pounds you will find the most effective and healthiest way is by sensible dieting combined with exercise. An added advantage of exercising is the cosmetic effect. When the fat disappears, skin begins to sag. The toning exercises for the arms and thighs I describe in Chapter 4 help ward off that unpleasant scraggy look.

Many people still believe that the best way to lose weight is to cut down on eating and to some extent this is true. After all, if you use up 2500 calories a day and eat food worth 3500 calories the excess 1000 calories will be stored as fat. It has been proved, however, that people

Height		Small frame		Medium frame		Large frame	
ft in	(cm)	lb	kg	lb	kg	lb	kg
5 1	(155)	112–120	(51–54)	118–129	(54–59)	126–141	(57–64)
5 2	(157)	115–123	(52–56)	121–133	(55–60)	129–144	(59–65)
5 3	(160)	118–126	(54–57)	124–136	(56–62)	132–148	(60–67)
5 4	(163)	121–129	(55–58)	127–139	(58–63)	135–152	(61–69)
5 5	(165)	124–133	(56–60)	130–143	(59–65)	138–156	(63–71)
5 6	(168)	128–137	(58–62)	134–147	(61–67)	142–161	(64–73)
5 7	(170)	132–141	(60–64)	138–152	(63–69)	147–166	(67–75)
5 8	(173)	136–145	(62–66)	142–156	(64–71)	151–170	(68–77)
5 9	(175)	140–150	(63–68)	146–160	(66–73)	155–174	(70–79)
5 10	(178)	144–154	(65–70)	150–165	(68–75)	159–179	(72–81)
5 11	(180)	148–158	(67–72)	154–170	(70–77)	164–184	(74–83)
6 0	(183)	152–162	(69–74)	158–175	(72–80)	168–189	(76–86)
6 1	(185)	156–167	(71–76)	162–180	(74–82)	173–194	(78–88)
6 2	(188)	160–171	(73–78)	167–185	(76–84)	178–199	(81–90)
6 3	(190)	164–175	(74–80)	172–190	(78–86)	182–204	(83–92)

Weight table for men aged 25 and over (in indoor clothing)

Height		Small frame		Medium frame		Large frame	
ft in	(cm)	lb	kg	lb	kg	lb	kg
4 8	(142)	92–98	(42–44)	96–107	(44–49)	104–119	(47–54)
4 9	(145)	94–101	(43–46)	98–110	(45–50)	106–122	(48–55)
4 10	(147)	96–104	(44–47)	101–113	(46–51)	109–125	(49–57)
4 11	(150)	99–107	(45–48)	104–116	(47–53)	112–128	(51–58)
5 0	(152)	102–110	(46–50)	107–119	(48–54)	115–131	(52–59)
5 1	(155)	105–113	(48–51)	110–122	(50–55)	118–134	(53–60)
5 2	(157)	108–116	(49–53)	113–126	(51–57)	121–138	(55–63)
5 3	(160)	111–119	(50–54)	116–130	(53–59)	125–142	(57–64)
5 4	(163)	114–123	(52–56)	120–135	(54–61)	129–146	(58–66)
5 5	(165)	118–127	(53–58)	124–139	(56–63)	133–150	(60–68)
5 6	(168)	122–131	(55–59)	128–143	(58–65)	137–154	(62–70)
5 7	(170)	126–135	(57–61)	132–147	(60–67)	141–158	(64–72)
5 8	(173)	130–140	(59–63)	136–151	(62–69)	145–163	(66–74)
5 9	(175)	134–144	(61–65)	140–155	(63–70)	149–168	(68–76)
5 10	(178)	138–148	(63–67)	144–159	(65–72)	153–173	(69–78)

Weight table for women aged 25 and over (in indoor clothing) (For women aged between 18 and 25 subtract 1 lb (½ kilo) for each year under 25)

have variable rates at which they burn up food (metabolic rates) and that regular exercise can help to speed up the rate considerably, not just during exercise but also for a period afterwards. The length of time depends on how vigorously you exercise. It also seems that people who drastically reduce their food intake lower their metabolic rate and so without exercise their weight loss may in fact slow down.

A calorie is the heat needed to raise the temperature of 1 gram of water by 1°C. Your body burns calories for energy:

About 2 calories per minute:	Sitting or standing still
About 3 calories per minute:	Washing and shaving, reading, driving, cooking, writing letters, laying the table, dusting, sewing
About 4 calories per minute:	typing, knitting, walking, light gardening
About 5 calories per minute:	housework, painting the house, walking upstairs
About 7 calories per minute:	playing cricket or baseball, bicycling, playing tennis, scrubbing floors
About 10 calories per minute:	jogging, swimming for pleasure, carrying heavy objects, making love, looking after a demanding child
Up to 20 calories per minute:	taxing exercises such as gym classes, competitive swimming, ballet classes, weightlifting, heavy gardening; football, running, squash; heavy work (on a building site, road work); boxing

The calorie-burning rate of some normal daily activities

How does exercise burn off calories? During thirty minutes of vigorous activity about 450 calories may be burned up – but another 550 calories are likely to be used up over the next day or two because of those thirty minutes. The good point for the overweight is obviously that they are likely to lose weight if a sensible eating plan and exercise routine are put into action.

Remember, though, that because of this continued higher metabolic rate you may have slightly lower blood sugars than normal for several hours and so it is wise to watch out for hypo symptoms until you have adjusted to a regular routine including exercise.

How much should you eat before, during and after exercise?

This is the million dollar question. After all, there are so many varying factors involved. It is perhaps easier to give advice to non insulin-dependent diabetics. Insulin reactions are not normally a problem for them, though occasionally people who take tablets may feel slight effects of low blood sugar and they need to deal with these in the same way as the insulin-dependents do. If you have experienced any hypo symptoms during exercise it would be wise to have an extra 10 g of carbohydrate before exercising and to keep a fast-acting glucose or sugar food close to hand.

For the insulin-dependent I cannot prescribe any exact amount of food to be taken. Unfortunately, like many aspects of looking after diabetes, trial and error is the key to the right formula for each individual. Let me give my own carbohydrate intake to show you what I mean.

On days when I am teaching for one hour mid-morning, I normally have an extra 10 g of long-acting carbohydrate with my breakfast such as wholemeal bread or bran-type cereal, plus 10 g of carbohydrate just before I exercise, in the form of a bran biscuit or fruit. If I need a little extra carbohydrate halfway through, I normally take it in the form of fruit juice or milk so that it is quickly and easily digested.

Within two hours of my class I eat a balanced lunch including protein (fish, eggs or meat), carbohydrates (potatoes, rice, pasta or bread) and vegetables or salad. More often than not I find it necessary to add 10 g of carbohydrate to my lunch to prevent a delayed insulin reaction following the morning's activity.

On days when I do two classes in the morning, I usually increase my breakfast by 15 g of carbohydrate and my pre-exercise snack to 15 g, as well as having an in-between class snack of 15 g of carbohydrate. Again, I have a little more carbohydrate than usual about two hours after the workout. On days when I am feeling particularly tired I may even need more than these amounts of carbohydrate with my mid-morning snack or at lunchtime.

But the best way to assess the amount you need is to experiment with your home monitoring tests:

7.30	test sugar pre-injection (blood or urine as usual)
7.45	breakfast (including 10 or 15 g extra carbohydrate; North America: eg, $^2/_3$ to 1 portion starchy foods)
10.00	pre-exercise test
	pre-exercise snack (10 or 15 g carbohydrate)
10.15–11.15	exercise, including 10 or 15 g instant carbohydrate snack
11.30	test sugar
12.30	lunch plus 10 or 15 g extra carbohydrate
16.00	final test and snack (10 or 15 g carbohydrate)

It should not be necessary to do this intense testing regularly, but it is worth trying on three or four occasions to make sure that you are maintaining your balance and not swinging the sugar pendulum too far either way. Discuss with your doctor what to do if the tests aren't within your target level.

In some books it is suggested that a small bar of chocolate is an ideal pre-exercise snack but I have found that by the end of an hour's good workout I have burned off this snack and am verging on a hypo. Long-acting, high-fibre foods will usually serve you better. They are digested more slowly and so the rise and fall of your blood sugars are more controlled.

I would advise any exerciser who feels hypo symptoms and needs to stop and eat some fast-acting carbohydrate to relax for at least ten to fifteen minutes afterwards until the carbohydrate has been absorbed and the body has fully adjusted. Don't try to continue exercising straight-away. Your reactions may still be a little delayed and unreliable, and you could in certain sports be a danger both to yourself and other people.

As a diabetic you will probably have access to a dietitian at the clinic or hospital you attend. It may be a good idea to discuss your carbohydrate intake for exercising with him or her if you find it difficult to achieve a comfortable balance.

How often and for how long should you exercise?

The answer is far from clear-cut because it depends on so many factors. Simple exercise like walking can be done for an hour or more every day, provided it causes no pains or strains. Playing squash or working out in a keep-fit group or gymnasium may, if overdone, be damaging to your health and to your diabetic routine.

The boom of keep-fit groups has encouraged many men and women to take up voluntary exercise at evening classes or in sports centres but often the outcome is that after each class their muscles ache and for the next day or two there are constant moans and groans, and then they do nothing until the next class when the same thing happens. This approach isn't beneficial and you are more likely to suffer from strains and injuries if you exercise at such infrequent intervals. It is wise to spread the amount you do over the week rather than cram hours of activity into the weekend or one evening and then do nothing during the rest of the week. It may be that you can fit in only one game or session of the type of activity you enjoy most in each week. In order to keep yourself fit enough to continue your energetic exercise, you must try to do some simple exercises or brisk walking on the other days.

With the aid of the exercises in Chapter 4 you should be able to do enough each day to keep you toned up between classes or games. If you travel to work by train, take advantage of the stairs rather than escalators or lifts. Try getting off the bus one stop before your normal one. You'll be surprised how just a few minutes' extra exercise each day will help you to get and keep fit.

What is the ideal amount of exercise that you should be doing?
Of course the answer varies greatly according to the individual but these hints should help you decide where to begin.

1. Exercise time includes walking, playing sports and any conscious form of physical activity (see Chapter 2).
2. As I said above, it is far better to spread three hours' exercise evenly over the week than to cram them into one Sunday session on the running track. As a diabetic it is sensible to be reasonably regular in the amount of exercise you do, especially when you begin. This is because different amounts at different times of day could mean daily alterations to your carbohydrate intake – if you can find only ten minutes a day, that's better than nothing. On days when you are not in the mood or are not feeling up to doing your exercise, remember to revert to your slightly lower carbohydrate allowance.

Five to twelve   Children are bound to include physical exercise in their daily routine without persuasion, but a minimum one hour a day of conscious exercise should be encouraged. This may be taken at school in the form of gym, sports or in the playground, or in after-school and weekend activities. I'm sure many children, diabetic or not, do as much as two to three hours a day physical activity. (Watching television does not constitute physical activity!)

Twelve to twenty   Surprisingly, many teenagers find every excuse to opt out of exercise, preferring more sedentary interests, but for diabetes' sake a minimum of an hour each day should be set aside for some conscious physical activity whether it is cycling, swimming, running, playing team games or dancing.

Twenty to thirty   Nowadays, people in this age group are often car-bound and do anything to avoid walking, so here again at least forty-five minutes a day of physical activity would go down well. Naturally many people in this age group are committed to their careers and families which can be very time consuming, but allowing forty-five minutes a day isn't very much to expect; it can be split into fifteen minutes in the morning and thirty minutes in the evening.

Thirty to forty-five   This is the time when you decide either to relax into middle age or regain lost youth. Don't be fanatical either way but do ensure that forty-five minutes each day is spent doing some conscious activity.

Forty-five to sixty There is normally little reason to slow down just because you've passed your forty-fifth birthday. Just say 'Many happy returns' and keep on exercising. Minimum, say fifteen minutes to begin with and if possible fifteen minutes twice a day – more if you're able.

Sixty plus At sixty you may be as active as when you were forty and as long as you are realistic you can carry on exercising. If you are a beginner at physical jerks after years of fairly sedentary living, start with just ten minutes a day and increase to ten minutes twice a day. Once again, if you feel fit and able you can build up to any amount you like within reason.

When should you stop exercising?

You may well ask, what are the signs of overdoing exercise? In general, it is safe to say that as long as your diabetic control is maintained (see pages 10–11) and you are not suffering from muscle, ligament or tendon strains or backache, or are generally unwell, then there is no reason why you shouldn't exercise.

One thing is for sure, *pain is warning* and as a general rule, when in pain, stop and rest.

Although we all speak about this pain or that one, actually defining pain is difficult, though any really persistent discomfort should be regarded as a warning. If you experience any sharp, piercing sensations anywhere or feelings of cramp, ease off the exercise for a while. You can go back to it after the strained muscles have stopped aching, but remember to begin again gradually.

If you continue having pains or cramps it may be wise to ask for some medical advice. Pains in the head or chest should be checked out if they start whenever you attempt exercise.

Foot cramp This is one of the more likely sources of trouble when you begin exercising. If you are inclined to have foot cramp anyway, it can be made worse by vigorous foot exercises. If you are caught by a sudden cramp, do some gentle relaxing and stretching to release the spasm. It should go away on its own within a few minutes. Once you know a certain exercise causes cramp, leave it out of your workout.

Breathing

Breathing is obviously a major aspect of exercise, yet often people are confused about the different ways they are told to breathe. People spend much time discussing deep and shallow breathing. For water sports there *are* right and wrong ways, but for most activities I put the main emphasis on even, regular breathing and trying to maintain a calm, rhythmic pace. You should aim for your own comfort and a regular breathing pace that suits you. Hurried, short breaths definitely make exercise harder work than necessary.

What time of day is best?

There are no set rules. Some people like to exercise early in the morning whilst others are happier to do it just before going to bed. As I've already said, it is sensible to keep to one time of the day, and as a diabetic, particularly if you are on insulin, it is better for you to exercise after your food and/or injection rather than beforehand. Vigorous exercise without sufficient insulin will raise blood sugars and upset your control.

Remember that strenuous activity continues to burn up energy for some time after you have actually stopped the exercise, so that your blood sugars will continue to fall steadily for the next hour or so. To prevent a hypoglycaemic attack, don't forget to eat a little extra long-acting carbohydrate (see page 19). It is particularly important to take this into account if you exercise before going to bed.

Where to exercise

1. For indoor exercising it is best to use an uncluttered room that is reasonably well ventilated. Draughts are not ideal ventilation, so don't fling open the windows before you begin. Make sure there's enough air coming into the room by leaving the door open. If you get very hot during the exercise you can open windows as you go. Close them as you slow down again and begin to feel colder.
2. If there is an open fire in the room, make sure that there is no chance of you actually falling into it, and remember that gas heaters give off some fumes which can be unpleasant during exercise.
3. If you live in an apartment and are intending to jog on the spot or skip, spare a thought for neighbours who live beneath you – don't decide to do it in your bedroom late at night.
4. Even if you have soft carpet flooring, use a mat or towel for exercises on the floor. This will prevent the fibres from irritating your skin and nose and you will be more comfortable.

What to wear

It is really quite unnecessary to spend a lot of money on special exercise clothes. Shoes should be your main concern and will be your main expenditure. All you need is an outfit that doesn't cramp your style, and several layers of it: old tee shirts and loose-fitting cotton trousers are perfectly all right if you don't want to go to the expense of a new track suit. You will need leg warmers and tights or track suit bottoms, or both, but these need not be expensive.

You should wear more than one layer of clothes when you work out for two reasons. First, the warmer your body is the less chance you have of pulling any muscles and second, it is miserable to exercise when you're cold. Even in spring and summer I wear woolly leg warmers over tights to maintain body heat in my calves and ankles – the areas most susceptible to sprains and strains. As soon as the weather cools I wear a leotard, tee shirt, track suit bottoms or sweat pants and leg warmers; and the full track suit as the winter settles, until I am warm enough to take off the top. My students very rarely see my legs in cool weather! Remember, we diabetics do have a tendency to feel the cold, particularly in the hands and feet, so wrap up!

Clothes to avoid

1. Do not wear any clothes that restrict your movement or that might get caught up in furniture.
2. Take off jewellery; dangling earrings have a knack of latching on to woolly tops and necklaces can pull tight around your neck.
3. Flowing nightwear may whisk past a fire and set you alight, so if exercising before going to bed, wear perhaps some short pyjamas – but don't forget to keep warm.

Footwear

Don't ever exercise in bare feet. Diabetics are prone to foot infections which can lead to serious problems (see page 15), so always wear comfortable footwear which keeps its shape and allows your feet to breathe. Joggers, diabetic or not, are realizing the benefits of good footwear. Good jogging shoes are absolutely essential, even for those new to the activity.

When buying shoes it is wise to go to a sports shop where you will get proper assistance, rather than a fashion shop that does not specialize in sports shoes. You need proper ankle support and plenty of inner padding, especially under the heel. But avoid shoes with rough interior stitching as they can cause blisters.

If you intend to do any jogging you should get shoes with a heavy-grip rubber sole and leather or leather and nylon uppers that give proper ventilation. This type of shoe is also right for the indoor workout but do ensure that the soles are really non-slip if that's what you're buying them for.

Always wear absorbent woollen or cotton socks when wearing training shoes and if the shoes stretch after they have been worn in, add an inner sole. Finally, try to break in sports shoes for short periods rather than wearing them the first time for a whole tennis match or putting them on for your first keep-fit session.

Here are some tips to help you to keep your feet in top condition:

1. Heels: for women in particular, fashion is often the dictator, but frankly, high heeled stiletto-type shoes can only threaten the circulation, safety and shape of the foot and ankle. It is the people who normally wear high heels who are more likely to suffer injuries to their feet, simply because their Achilles tendon muscles (at the

rear of the heel) are unused to being stretched. If you usually wear high heels, before attempting any exercise always do the warm-up exercise specifically designed to stretch these muscles (see page 36).

2. Don't wear sports shoes regularly as casual shoes: you should change your footwear often so that your feet do not become too used to any one shape of shoe; and exercise shoes particularly should be given ample time to dry out after having been worn for a sweaty game of football or tennis.

3. Beware of swimming pools, sports hall floors and changing rooms: splinters and infections lurk in these places so keep your feet covered. It is wise to wear rubber or plastic sandals to the edge of the pool and in the showers.

4. If you have any foot problems, don't be afraid to seek professional advice. Diabetic clinics often have their own chiropodists who will check your feet and give useful advice. It is worth looking after your feet *now*, before the real problems appear. Prevention is better than cure!

5. Whenever you have some spare time, especially just after a bath or before going to bed, pamper your feet a little by massaging in some moisturizing lotion to keep the skin supple. At the same time don't forget to check for blisters, splinters or any infection.

2 DIFFERENT FORMS OF EXERCISE

In this book I describe a workout routine that can be followed more or less energetically by any diabetic according to ability. But my get fit is not the only type of exercise you are going to be doing.

It would be difficult for me to list all the activities that may be available to you but in this chapter I describe the most popular ones with guidance on their benefits and their relation to diabetes.

Conscious and unconscious exercise

Exercise can be broken down into two main types, conscious and unconscious. You may well ask what I mean by unconscious exercise; walking to work, doing the gardening or the home decorating can all be classed as unconscious. After all they are jobs that have to be done and in doing them you are using your muscles and burning up energy. Women have often told me that they get enough exercise from being housewives and mothers. The diabetic, particularly the insulin-dependent, should think carefully about these types of unconscious activity. Without preparation, an hour digging in the garden can lead to a hypoglycaemic attack. As well as eating a little extra carbohydrate before the activity (see page 19), remember to keep some glucose or instant carbohydrate on you just in case of a low blood sugar attack.

Undoubtedly an active life can provide enough strenuous exercise of the unconscious sort but conscious planned exercise gives more benefit, particularly because of its relaxing effect. Choosing a sport or activity like keep fit, golf or bowls may also involve you in meeting new people, and getting a break from your circle or family. It may get you out of doors in the fresh air and above all it will mean a complete change of environment which does wonders for releasing the tensions and stresses of everyday living.

Here are some points to bear in mind when you begin your active routine:

Unconscious exercise

Regular housework should not cause any problems for the diabetic. In fact, scrubbing and polishing floors, shopping or gardening will burn up those extra calories if you need to lose weight. But for the big spring clean or bout of decorating, take precautions against hypo attacks. Always set aside five minutes each hour for a well-deserved coffee break.

Conscious exercise

Walking This is one of the finest types of exercise for all ages. There's no need to load yourself up with extra carbohydrate for a one-mile jaunt or thirty minutes with the dog, but for day-long hikes, keep yourself stocked up with essential foods and never go off alone for long country walks without informing someone of your route and destination.

For the overweight, try walking instead of other types of transport whenever possible. This will burn off calories gently without straining the heart or muscles. Remember, sensible low-heeled and well-fitting walking shoes are essential.

Jogging This is one of the most fashionable fads in getting fit! Don't rush out and try to jog 3 miles (5 km) without preparation, but aim to build up distances gradually by walking and jogging intermittently. The overweight or over thirties should get approval from their doctor before starting jogging.

As this is a heart-strengthening exercise (aerobic) you will burn up calories at a particularly fast rate so testing your sugar regularly will be necessary to begin with (see page 19).

Running Like jogging this is an aerobic exercise, but more vigorous. Whether you are marathon running or lapping the school track for fun, learn to judge your sugar levels by monitoring them regularly and always keep instant carbohydrate available. Several diabetics have run in marathons that have been held over the last few years and they needed careful constant preparation for months in advance. Always begin your running programme with plenty of warm-up exercises (see Chapter 4).

For the overweight, running is likely to be too strenuous and should not be attempted until most of the excess weight is off.

Football, ball games and hockey All these team sports require maximum effort from each player and so your diabetes must be under perfect control and not become a burden on the team. If you are insulin-dependent, keep stocked up on carbohydrate and have a sugar check at half-time breaks. Fast-acting carbohydrate such as a glass of fresh orange juice and a bran biscuit is the type of food to eat at half-time, not a cheese sandwich, which is difficult to digest.

Dancing and keep-fit workouts There is a big fashion now in keeping fit to music, whether in discotheques or in dance studios. Take advantage of the wide variety of dance-type activities but remember that when you begin you cannot expect to get through the classes as easily as people who have been attending regularly. Be cautious of huge classes without room to move and of classes where the teachers offer no, or very little, explanation and demonstration.

Tell the teacher of your condition just in case of problems, particularly if you are on insulin, and don't be embarrassed to eat some fast-acting carbohydrate half-way through. Better that than a hypo! If you suffer or have suffered from non-diabetic problems such as back strain, knee problems or headaches, remember to let the instructor know that too.

Wear comfortable training shoes for keep fit (see page 24), and dance shoes or tennis shoes for dancing, rather than going barefoot.

If you go out dancing with friends in the evening, don't forget to take the same precautions – eat a little extra carbohydrate first and keep a fast-acting type with you. It's easy to get carried away when the beat is good!

Squash   This is one of the most strenuous sports, even if played at beginner's level. There is no reason why you should not play if you are otherwise fit and not too overweight, but keep a check on your sugar and try to play people of your own ability. Remember to let your partner know of your condition (particularly if on insulin). Because the game is very fast and unpredictable you can easily feel confused and light-headed and may not notice hypo symptoms developing. I have known of insulin-dependent diabetics coming off court with fairly normal blood sugars and within twenty minutes being very hypo, because such strenuous activity goes on burning up energy for a while after the action has stopped. Be prepared for this delayed action by eating a little extra carbohydrate after a hard game.

Avoid muscle strain by warming up thoroughly before going on court as well as finishing off with a few slowing down exercises.

Swimming   For diabetics there are some important rules for swimming. In swimming pools: tell someone, preferably a lifeguard, you are diabetic, and if you are insulin-dependent give that person some sugar to hold for you. People may think you're fooling around if you begin acting strangely due to a hypo.

The sea: never swim far out alone and without sugar. Liquid carbohydrate can be carried in a small plastic bottle around your waist, but don't forget a high tide or rough sea can draw you out to sea quickly and however well you can swim, a hypo could be fatal if not treated.

Sea swimmers should wear plastic or rubber footwear as protection against sea nasties like prickly urchins, coral or jellyfish.

Bearing all that in mind, swimming is an excellent form of exercise, both as a heart-strengthener and a toner and stretcher. Backache sufferers and often disabled people benefit particularly from swimming in heated indoor pools since the water carries body weight quite effortlessly – especially if it's salt water.

3 EXERCISE FOR DIFFERENT AGES

In the last chapter, I gave some idea of the pitfalls to look out for when going in for different types of exercise. Of course exercise varies according to your age, and here I describe some of the special problems for each different group.

Under fives

Diabetes in toddlers under five years old is far from common – there are under one in a thousand in the UK – but in nearly all cases it is controlled by insulin injections. Looking after a diabetic child is often a big worry for the parents to start with. They have to know how to teach their child to cope with the condition and it is they who must help instil confidence.

Diabetic toddlers should be encouraged to be as active as any other child, having swimming lessons with mothers and going to playgroups. Parents will have to ensure that their baby has been properly fed before any extra activity and it is also wise to let crèche supervisors or activity helpers know about the child's condition and how to cope.

School years

Most schools accept diabetic children and it is important that they are not left out of any school activities, especially sports and outings. There is bound to be plenty of physical activity for the child once he or she begins school and the parents must tell the teachers of the special needs that the child has since they may not know much about diabetes – for example, to ensure that there is enough carbohydrate to hand. Check with staff too that your child gets enough of the right food at school meals. Generally though, even five-year-olds are amazingly sensible when they have to learn to cope with the condition.

Nowadays most diabetics over eight manage to do their own injections, test their own sugar levels and count their own carbohydrate intake.

The British Diabetic Association and parallel organizations in North America and Australia (see Useful Addresses) have helped thousands of young children cope with their own condition by offering holidays which are specially designed to teach them control. These breaks usually include plenty of sporting activities such as hiking, swimming, canoeing, rock-climbing and camping, which apart from being fun are a good way for them to get to know their carbohydrate requirements while exercising.

School holidays Insulin and food requirements will probably alter during long school vacations. This is largely due to the change in your routine and because you may have the occasional extra treat of ice cream or chocolate during the holidays.

Keeping to a set routine during the holidays is difficult. Try to take some exercise, even if it is only going for a walk. That way you will not be making too big a change in your blood sugar control.

Teenagers
This a time that is full of changes, both physical and mental, and these go hand in hand with new social activities like discos and parties and you may be among friends who start to drink and smoke. It is a time when you are likely to experience hypo attacks unless you remember to think ahead.

Points to remember

- Disco dancing is great exercise but you may need extra food.
- Smoking does you no good.
- Drinking should be checked – the sugar content of some alcoholic drinks will interfere with your blood sugar balance. Don't substitute alcohol for other sugar in your diet.
- Sexual activity is generally very physical and emotional and tends to lower the blood sugar. Eating may seem a ridiculous point to have to think about, but you should get used to the idea of making provision, and talking openly with your partner about it.

Marriage and parenthood
Diabetics free of complications are no longer normally discouraged from marriage or motherhood now that the risks to the mother and baby can be minimized by careful control.

Exercise should play a major part in helping both parents relax and prepare for the birth. Fathers no longer take the back seat and in many cases they choose to be present at the birth. The father can learn to be of great assistance during the labour period by helping the mother do the exercises and breathing that she has been taught.

There are special antenatal (or prenatal) clinics for the diabetic mother that give the necessary dietary and other advice during pregnancy and she will make regular visits to the clinic for check-ups. Some clinics hold special exercise classes that the father can also attend.

How much exercise during pregnancy? If you want to take up an exercise routine during pregnancy you must check with your doctor that you are capable of it. During the first few months strenuous exercise should be avoided, particularly at the time that a period would normally be due since it is then that miscarriages are most likely to occur. Changes

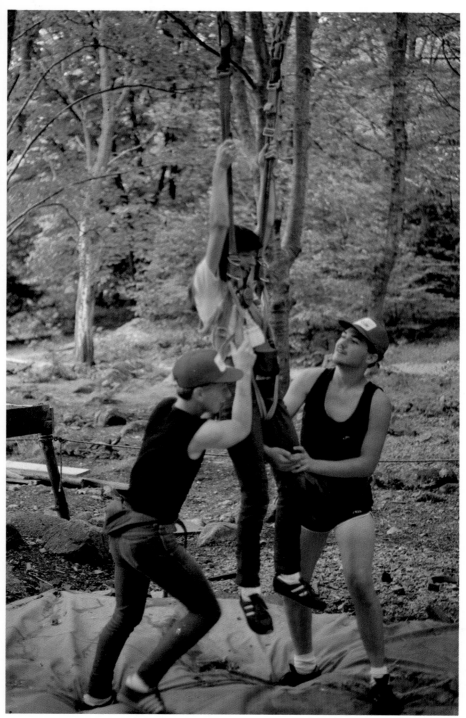

Young diabetics learning to land after a forty-foot fixed parachute jump: one of the many exciting activities they are taught on special courses.

in the blood sugars due to the pregnancy are common in the first month. If you suspect or know you are pregnant, you should restrict your exercise to the gentle routine I outline on pages 92–9. If you are planning other forms of exercise, swimming and walking are fine, but not tennis or squash, or similar vigorous sports.

The diabetic mother   It is generally considered that the birth of a baby, particularly the first child, is going to be the finest and most wonderful period in your life, and all being well it will be. Don't be surprised though if the first few weeks, and even months, aren't quite the perfect joy you expected them to be. Having a baby is tiring and after the birth you may be at quite a low ebb. Your diabetes will be watched very carefully by all concerned. It is also up to you and your partner to ensure that you spend sufficient time caring for your own well-being as well as the baby's. Getting back into good physical shape doesn't mean strict dieting and rigorous exercise but allowing rest periods during the day, getting plenty of air, doing gentle exercise and eating a well-balanced diet of fresh, wholesome foods. The extra weight will come off fairly quickly and regular low-key exercise will help firm up the sagging abdomen and pelvic muscles (see page 83).

Don't rush to your nearest keep-fit class before being checked out by your doctor. I've occasionally had new mothers turn up at my classes with three-week-old babies and have had to send them home again. Patience is necessary in these early days.

After a few months you will settle down to a fairly regular routine and be feeling more fit. Now is the time to get out and get back into the swing. You can go back to any sport you want or join a keep-fit class. More and more groups are setting up babysitting facilities to allow mothers a little time to themselves. The break for an hour or so will be rewarding and refreshing, so don't feel guilty. Do, on the other hand, check that you are happy with the facilities in the day centre and that the helpers seem responsible and caring.

The middle years
The majority of diabetics will discover their condition during middle age and many of them will also be at least a little overweight. Exercise is especially important for non insulin-dependent diabetics. It will speed up weight loss which in turn will help to keep the blood sugars controlled, and it will firm the figure. But it is imperative to get the okay from your doctor before you begin your exercise programme.

If you are an insulin-dependent diabetic it is as important now as ever to keep up a regular fitness programme. Many people slip into a slower pace of life during these less hectic years and their sugar levels may get a little out of control due to lack of regular activity. This is when the risk of diabetic complications may set in, so keep regular exercise as part of your routine and don't feel threatened by 'middle age'. It should be a prime time in your life! You will find plenty of opportunities for new activity at this stage, when your children are leaving home and becoming independent; you may also be retired – in any case, you are likely to have spare time on your hands which you can put to good use. Obviously if you are starting after years of relative inactivity, you must begin with great care, and preferably with your doctor's consent if you have any doubts.

If you have not been sporty during your twenties and thirties, you should take up activities such as swimming, dancing, walking, cycling, golf or gardening rather than squash or vigorous workouts. For starters, try doing some of the warm-up exercises in Chapter 4. Now that your home life may not be quite so frantic as when the family were younger, you should be able to spare about forty-five minutes each day – split up into two or three separate sessions – for exercise and relaxation. Remember a few minutes' daily exercise is far better than one long hard session only once a week.

Getting older

Diabetes is increasingly common in older people, more so than in the middle-aged (about 20 per cent of older people have it). It is never very easy to accept or to learn how to cope with the condition and after sixty it may be hard to convince yourself, when you have just been diagnosed as diabetic, that you can take up an active, healthy life. But don't give up. As long as you have a little mobility there are exercises that you can do too. Gentle walking, ballroom dancing or gardening are marvellous sorts of exercise, as are activities such as handicrafts and singing, which although not physically demanding are great fun. There have been very successful marathon runners in the last few years who have been well into their seventies and even their eighties. Of course asking you to consider marathon running would be ridiculous and you shouldn't try this sort of energetic exercise without having trained all your life. But a daily routine of suitable exercise is as important for keeping yourself in trim and your blood sugar normal as it is for younger diabetics.

Even if it is very difficult for you to arrange to do regular out-of-doors activity, there are many mobility exercises that can be done in your own home and even in the comfort of your own chair (I indicate these in the workout described in Chapter 4).

4 THE HOME EXERCISE ROUTINE

Having read the first part of this book, you will realize that it's up to you to assess your own fitness and what your requirements for exercise are. As a diabetic you will be used to monitoring your health, so it's less of a worry for you to take decisions about starting a new get-fit programme than for people who haven't any experience of checking themselves. All the same, if you're ever in doubt about the levels you're aiming for, I'm sure your doctor or clinic will be only too glad to advise you.

Benefits of the indoor workout
Whatever your age and ability, the following workout will have something suitable for you. The benefits of making a daily workout part of your exercise plan are enormous: it costs you nothing; very little time is needed either to prepare or to do the exercises; you can choose the time of day that is best for you.

Music
If you are anything like me, you will enjoy doing your exercises to music as long as it has a rhythm that is regular and neither too hurried nor too slow. You can experiment with different sorts. Music is often used for relaxation therapy, so clearly combining it with exercise makes the whole business of getting fit more fun and more beneficial than ever.

Preparing for your exercise routine

Due to the recent interest in fast workout-type exercise, many people think it will be good for them only if it makes them sweat and it hurts. It is now being seen that many injuries, both short and long-term, have been caused by people exercising too much too soon rather than building up gradually and patiently. As exercise is an aid to a better life, don't rush – there is no need. Slow, gentle stretching can be just as good if not more so, for toning and firming muscle and awakening the body and mind.

Yoga-type exercise has been around for many years and though it is not everyone's idea of a workout it does provide flexibility, mental well-being and mobility with very few reports of injury. The exercises in this workout do not fall into either the yoga or aerobic category but are based on all manner of movement, stretching and toning which should help you both physically and mentally.

Here is a list of points to remember before you start your new exercise routine.

1. Read through the whole exercise section first, studying the illustrations, before attempting anything.
2. For the first three or four attempts you can follow the whole routine as long as you begin gently and aren't getting too tired, but only do the minimum of repeats suggested. When you are feeling perfectly comfortable you can gradually build up the repetitions. Don't jump from four to sixteen in one go.
3. If any exercise is painful, and you are sure that you are following my instructions correctly, leave it out. Not every exercise is suitable for everyone. The most important thing about a regular exercise programme is the long-term benefits to both mind and body; over-energetic spurts of activity will probably result only in aches and pains and put you off (the can't be bothered syndrome).
4. Remember that the warm-up exercises are absolutely essential and on days when your time is very limited, the warm-up alone will be of benefit to you.
5. Always finish with at least some cool-down exercises.
6. Everyone has good and bad days. Don't be upset if one day you are unable to do as much as you were doing the previous day. Take it easy and try again the next day.
7. Always wear warm clothes, including leg warmers or track suit bottoms, for the warm-up stretches. If you begin to boil over then at least you can take off some clothing, but if you start wearing only the bare essentials, you are more likely to pull and strain muscles early on.
8. Women who wear high-heels should put on flat shoes at least one hour before starting so as not to over-stretch the Achilles tendon in the warm-up.
9. Don't stop too long between exercises or you'll find you lose body heat and muscles may begin to seize up.
10. As with non-diabetics, viruses, colds, flu and tummy upsets are generally quite exhausting and the body usually takes a week or two to get back to normal. Don't force yourself to do a long, hard workout if you haven't been well; your body does need time to replenish its deficiencies. When you feel better, remember to go back a step or two in the number of repetitions you try. Being less active, even for a week or two, gives the muscles a chance to relax and muscle strength must be rebuilt slowly. This is an important point for everyone, not only diabetics.

35

A final reminder: have you thought about your blood sugar, and if so, have you eaten sufficient carbohydrate to last you through this extra activity? Don't forget to have some fast-acting carbohydrate such as glucose tablets, orange juice or biscuits readily available just in case you have an unexpected hypo.

Note: Exercises marked with an asterisk * are suitable for the chair-bound and less mobile.

The warm-up

The warm-up is the most vital part of any strenuous activity, whether it is indoor exercises, cycling or preparing for a football or tennis match. Though the weather may be hot or the room heated, if your muscles have been rested they will need to be gently stretched in preparation for activity. For the diabetic, doing everything to prevent tendon and muscle strain is particularly important since putting yourself out of action is likely to upset your diabetic control.

The Achilles tendon stretch, *below*, and *right*, the ankle stretch

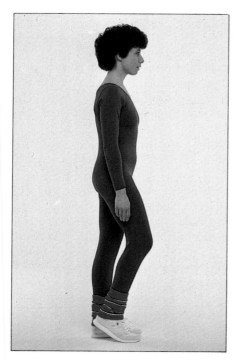 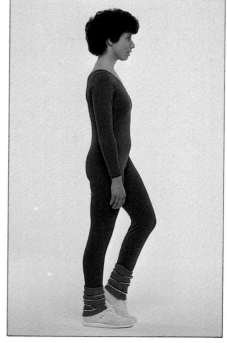

The Achilles tendon stretch

Stand with feet close together, hands and arms by your sides. Relax shoulders, neck, face. Lift one heel gently off the floor and slowly lower it down again whilst lifting the other heel off the floor. Try and work the muscles through to the foot and be careful not to bounce from one to another (which can damage your tendons) but to control gently the lift and lower stretch.

How many should you do? Because this initial stretch is so important, whatever your age or fitness level you should do at least twelve exchanges and up to about thirty once you are in practice. Aim to keep a steady rhythm to loosen and warm up for the following exercise.

The ankle stretch*

This is another essential warm-up exercise and can be done by chair-bound people too.

Stand with feet close together, or sit comfortably. Lift one foot off the floor, circle the ankle to the right several times, then make the same number of rotations to the left. Change to the other foot and repeat.

How many should you do? Start with three rotations each way with each foot and build up to six.

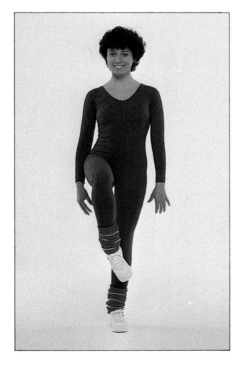 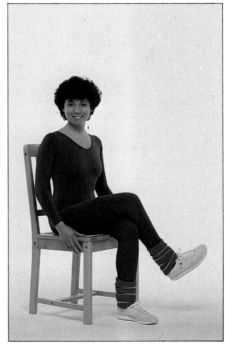

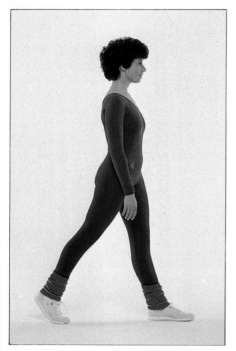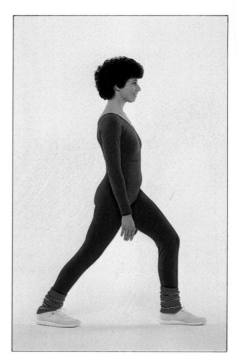

The calf muscle stretch

The calf muscle stretch
To begin with, stand with feet close together. Place the right foot about 2 to 3 ft (0.75 to 1 m) behind the left; only the toes of the right foot should be on the floor. Gently bend the front knee and move the right heel gently down towards the floor. You should certainly not aim to touch the floor for the first three or four bounces and don't force it after that.

So that you don't end up lop-sided, always do the same amount of exercising on each leg.

How many should you do? For all ages and abilities, between ten and fifteen slow and gentle bounces on each leg to ensure that the muscles have been well stretched, minimizing the chance of strains or sprains later in the routine.

Stretching

Now that you've warmed up and your muscles are loosened, you're ready for the big stretch.

One of the greatest causes of absence from work in the Western world is back trouble. The main reason is that we abuse our natural posture by sitting in incorrectly designed furniture and pay too little attention to our walking, working and sleeping positions. This problem may have little direct association with diabetes but bad posture can harm our general well-being. As well as looking unattractive it undoubtedly leads to tension of muscle groups which in turn may result in backache, neck strain or headaches. These exercises will do untold good by stretching your back and making you conscious of the proper way to stand. You can also try them sitting if you are chair-bound.

Basic posture (wrong and right)

Stand with your feet a little apart. Keep your weight off your heels so that you feel it is towards the front of your feet. Pull your tummy muscles in, lift your ribcage out of your waist, giving height to your body, but keep your shoulders relaxed. Let your hands and arms rest by your sides and keep your neck long. Look straight ahead and try to breathe calmly and gently.

Check your posture in a mirror and aim for the good tall position (*right*).

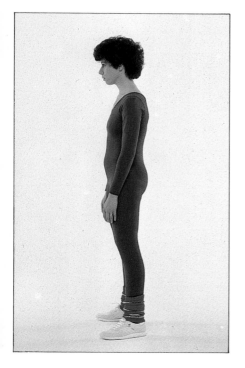
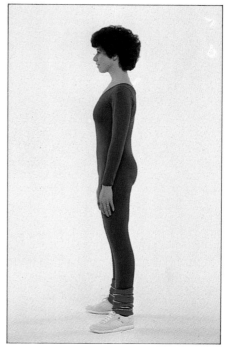

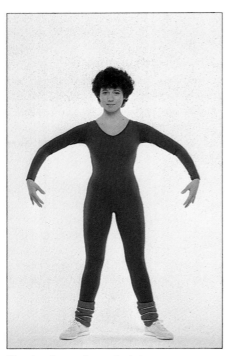
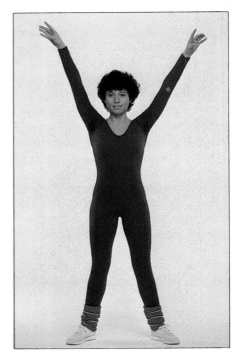

The basic posture stretch

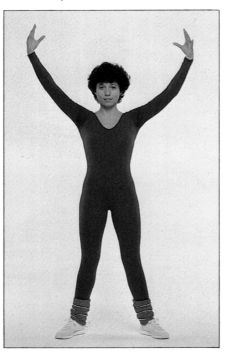
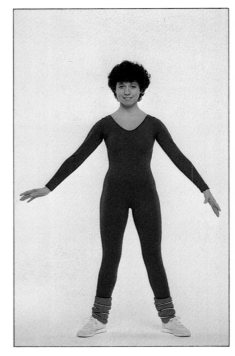

Basic posture stretch*

You can also do this stretch by itself, any time, when you feel the need for a good stretch.

Standing (or sitting) in the basic position, breathe in to the count of four and whilst doing so, lift your arms slowly out and above your head, keeping shoulders down and relaxed. Exhale and slowly lower the arms again, also to the count of four. Repeat this exercise at least four times.

The monkey swing

Stand with your feet a little apart, in the basic posture position. Lift your arms up to your head, and reach up first with the right and then with the left hand, feeling a stretch from your waist and stomach muscles. Now bend your knees a little and swing your arms down and up again, and swing once more down and up, before returning to the

The monkey swing

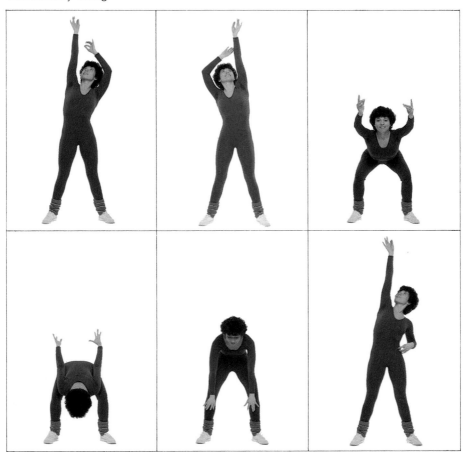

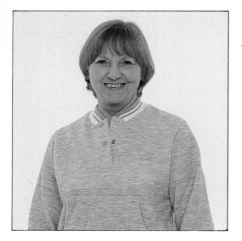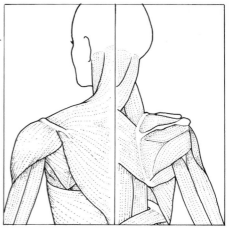

(*Left*) Smile: it's so simple but so effective. (*Right*) The different layers of muscle in the neck and shoulders, where tension can occur.

standing position with your arms above your head ready to repeat the exercise.

How many should you do? Beginners, start with three and build up to six. Fairly fit, start with five and build up to ten. Even fitter, start with six and build up to fifteen.

Face, neck, head and shoulders

These exercises are particularly helpful in reducing tension, stresses and anxieties. Undue stress doesn't go very well with diabetes and can cause erratic changes in blood sugars, as can emotional upset, illness and unplanned changes in physical activity (see Chapter 1). Whenever you are feeling tense, try the following exercises a few times.

This type of exercise is also ideal for chair-bound or partially disabled folk as well as the elderly who may be less fit.

My favourite one seems to work almost without fail, and is so easy. Smile! As you are reading this, just smile! If your smile is a sincere effort you will almost instantly feel brighter and less tense. It must be worth a try!

Tension is most commonly felt in the neck and shoulders and by sedentary office workers and craftsmen in particular; long periods of concentration can lead to hunched muscles in the upper vertebrae of the spine and muscles in the shoulders, resulting in headaches and general aches and pains.

Head and shoulder movement*
Either sit or stand comfortably with your hands and arms quite loose

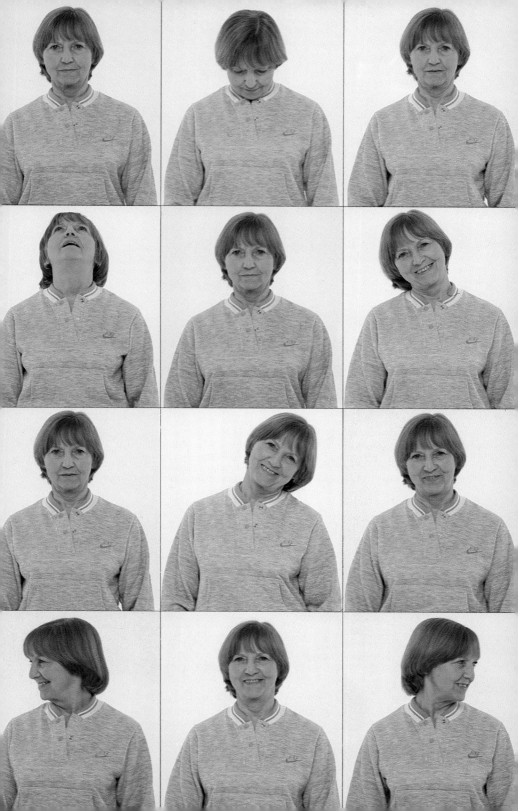

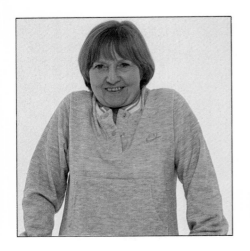 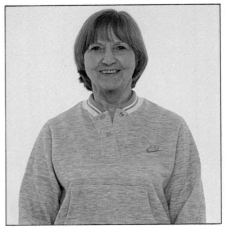

Shoulder lifts: this is a good exercise for tired or tense office workers and drivers.

by your sides. Let your head roll forward on to your chest, relax for two seconds and lift up to look ahead. Then let your head flop back, letting your mouth fall open, again holding the position for two seconds and returning to the middle position. With the same timing, let your head flop to each shoulder. Always return to the middle before going to the next position. Head to right, then to middle and then to left.

Shoulder lifts*
Great for releasing tension: sitting or standing, lift both shoulders to touch your ear lobes, hold for two seconds then let them relax.

Shoulders*
Sitting or standing with your shoulders relaxed: pull both shoulder blades back together and hold for two seconds. Then return to the relaxed position. Now gently pull your shoulders forward and together, opening the shoulder blades, and then relax back to the central position.

How many should you do? Do all these exercises at least once, and build up to eight repetitions.

Circulation for fingers, arms and hands

Circulation problems are most common in the feet and the hands. The same rules of keeping the skin supple and free of blisters and infections apply for your hands as for your feet (see Chapter 1) and the following exercises will help to maintain a good blood flow.

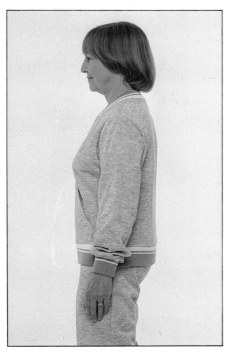
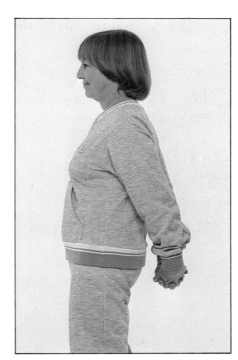

The shoulder exercise: for maximum stretch, straighten your elbows.

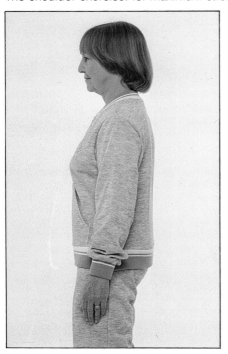
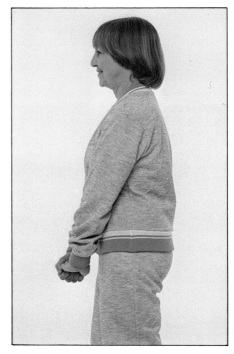

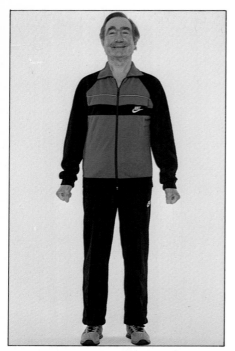
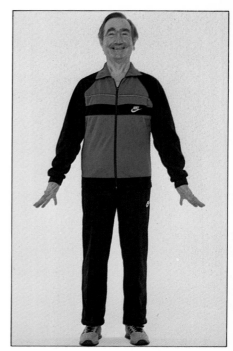

Fist clenching: in cold weather particularly this exercise will really help to improve circulation.

Fist clenching*
Sit or stand in a comfortable position with arms out by your sides, shoulders and face relaxed. (Don't forget to smile.) Slowly clench the fists and hold for two seconds, then release the fingers and stretch the hand out for two seconds.

How many should you do?   Repeat just a few times to begin with and build up to fifteen clenches.

Piano playing*
Even if you can't play the piano, this exercise is simple and effective – especially in cold weather – and can be done anywhere. Pretend there is a piano keyboard on your lap, and practise, one finger pressing a key at a time. First thumb, then index finger, forefinger, middle, and last the little finger. Repeat, starting with the little finger first.

How many should you do?   Start with a couple of repeats for each hand and build up to eight each.

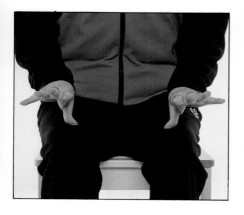
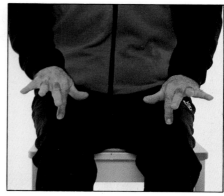
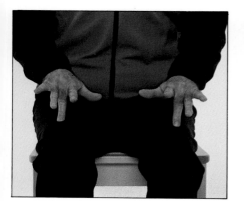
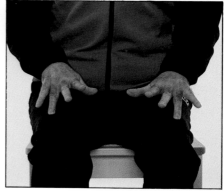
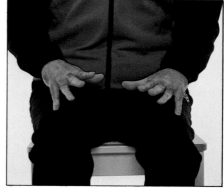

Piano playing: stretch each finger as much as you can to get the full benefit of this exercise.

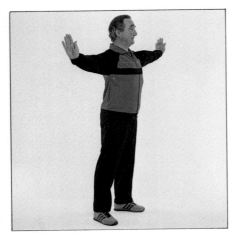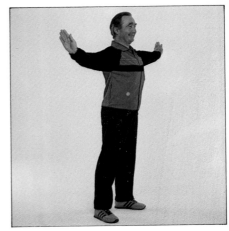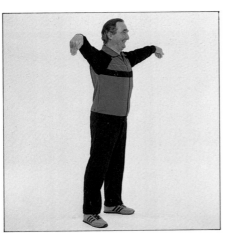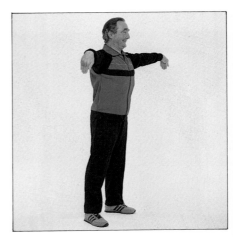

Arm circling: try to circle right from the shoulder.

Arm circling

Do this exercise to music – it's much easier and more enjoyable that way. It firms up flabby arms as well as helping circulation.

Stand with feet a little apart and arms out to the sides. Remember to keep your face relaxed, shoulders relaxed, tummy in and most of your weight forward, off your heels. Are you still breathing evenly? Comfortable? Okay, just circle your arms with straight elbows making small circles four times backwards with the hands flexed followed by four circles forwards with the hands pointing down. This exercise can be tiring and you should take rests by lowering your arms for fifteen seconds or so in between each set of circles until you have sufficient strength in the upper arms not to have to rest. As an alternative, simply hold out your arms and rotate, first palms upwards, then palms downwards.

How many should you do? Begin by circling backwards and forwards just twice, increasing the repetitions every two days up to sixteen each way.

The penguin stretch
Stand with feet apart, arms down by your sides and flex your hands so that your fingertips are at right angles to your body. Keeping the elbows locked into a straight position, raise your arms above your head so the fingertips touch, then gently lower them right down to your sides again.

The penguin stretch: keep both shoulders down and relaxed.

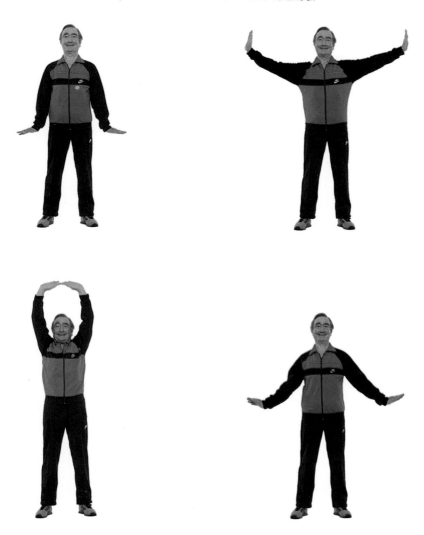

When doing this exercise, keep most of your weight off the heels and make sure that you are not pulling back when your arms meet. They should be a little in front of your head. Reason? So that you don't strain your lower back.

How many should you do?   Beginners, three to five; fairly fit, six to twelve; the even fitter, start with six and increase to twenty.

Toe, foot and ankle exercises

The nice part about these exercises is that most of them can also be done while you are sitting down, maybe watching the television or listening to music.

Choose your most comfortable position for ankle circling.

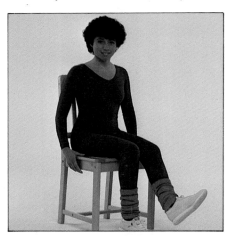
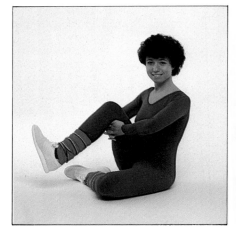

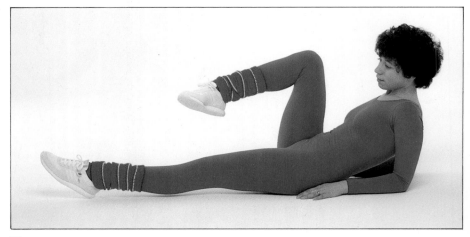

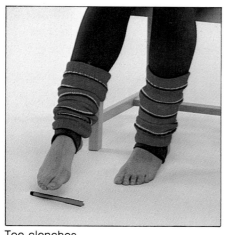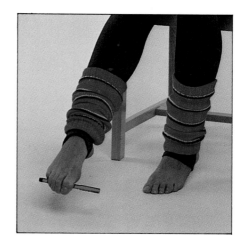

Toe clenches

Ankle circles*
Circle each foot about six times in each direction and then relax.

Toe clenches*
As well as helping circulation these are particularly good for strengthening the tendon and help fallen arches.

First remove your shoes! Then place a pencil or clean tissue on the floor and try to pick it up with your toes. Gradually move it a few inches away from its original place.

How many should you do?   Begin with two repetitions for each foot and gradually build up to six.

Pointing and flexing*
Either sitting or standing, lift one foot off the ground and point your

Pointing and flexing

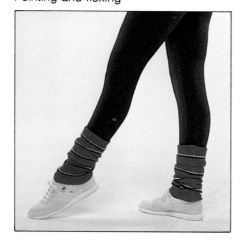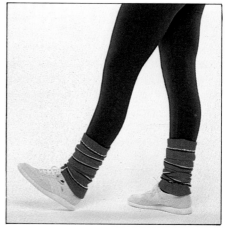

toes, feeling a stretch along the front of your leg. Then flex the foot so that you are stretching your heel and the stretch is now at the back of your leg.

How many should you do?   Point and flex each foot just four to six times to begin with and gradually increase to twelve times.

Note: If you suffer from foot cramp, this and the last exercise might bring it on, so eliminate them from your workout, if necessary. If you do get cramp, see my advice for relieving it on page 22.

Suppleness: trunk exercises

These are wonderful exercises for keeping everyone trim, but I find people over forty are especially pleased with the results. You must have heard people grumbling about their bodies feeling old and stiff. The truth is we expect to slow down and stiffen up with age and so we often don't do very much about it. But those common complaints of arthritis, rheumatism and bad backs are not directly linked with diabetes and if you take care of your body from an early age, there is little reason why you should stiffen up.

Overweight people often think being supple is associated only with slim, little people, but if you are trying to lose weight you will be surprised at just how supple you can be as you try to help your body adapt to its new shape.

The nice point about these exercises is that they are not fast and tiring. Done alone, they will not burn up too much sugar but as it is essential always to do the warm-up exercises beforehand, ensure that you have a reasonably good sugar level before you begin, and some instant carbohydrate to hand, just in case!

The spine
There are so many people who suffer from backache and neck problems that I am dividing these exercises into two sections, the first for good backs, and the second a few relaxation poses that may help to relieve pain in aching backs. Be cautious about exercising if you are suffering from back pain and if in any doubt, consult your doctor first.

The ripple
Stand with your feet a little apart and knees slightly bent; arms and hands relaxed just behind your thighs. Slowly bend your knees, keeping your heels on the floor, and let your chest roll out over your knees. When you are as low as you can be, let your head flop down and relax and let your arms relax in front of you too. Gently uncurl your body, keeping your head, neck, shoulders completely relaxed until you are

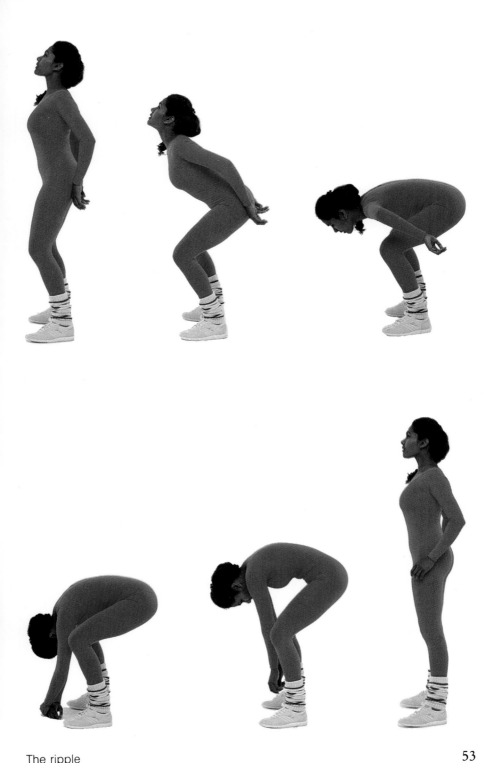

The ripple   53

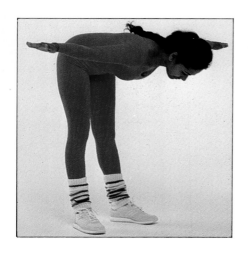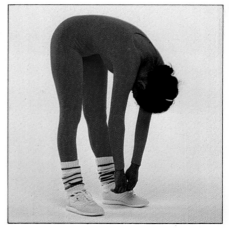

This exercise should be attempted only after a full warm-up since it places quite a strain on the calves and the hamstrings.

back to the standing position. Then slowly raise your head. To get the best effect from this exercise, try to go from one ripple to the next without more than two seconds' break in between – but do stop if you feel you have had enough.

How many should you do?   Beginners, just two to begin with and build up to four; fairly fit, begin with two and build up to six; even fitter, again begin with two and build up to six. Too many repetitions may make you feel dizzy.

The flat and arched back
Stand with your feet a little apart and with arms out to the side. Gently lower your head and spine so that your back is flat like a table top and your eyes are looking down to the floor. This is much harder than it sounds, but remember to keep most of your weight off the heels and make sure that you can feel a stretch at the back of your thighs. Hold the pose for two seconds. Then let your arms drop to your sides and arch your spine by letting your shoulders and head drop forward and pulling up from your tummy muscles. Hold for two seconds and then return to the flat back position. When you have had enough, let your body flop down in front of you, and very gently and slowly uncurl to a standing position.

How many should you do? Because this is quite a controlled and strenuous exercise it is not necessary to do too many. Three flat backs and three arches is an ample target for all abilities. If you enjoy doing this particular exercise you can repeat it later in the day, rather than double the number at one session.

Suppleness for problem backs

The majority of backaches are in the lower vertebrae and are often caused through poor posture or straining of the spine by carrying weights awkwardly. Long-term backaches can be due to wearing of the discs that separate the vertebrae or to trapped nerves. For this sort of trouble relief exercises and postures will be better than physical jerk type work-outs. The exercises below are not a cure for backaches but they can be very soothing. If in any doubt ask your doctor for his or her approval before trying them.

Relaxation poses

1. Lie on the floor with both knees pulled up to your chest and grasp your knees with your arms. Slowly and gently bring your forehead up towards your knees, hold the position for five seconds and then slowly relax your head down to the floor again.

2. Sit back on your heels, and place your arms by your side, lowering your head down towards the floor. Rest in this position for five to ten seconds and then slowly uncurl to a sitting position, still resting on your heels.

Try holding this position long enough to feel a complete stretch of the spine and neck.

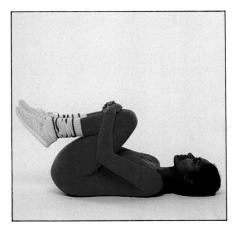
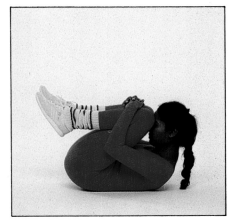

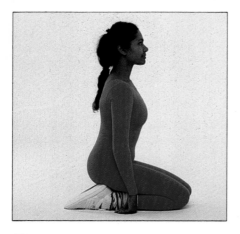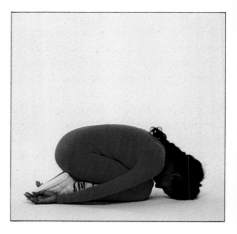

This exercise is commonly used in yoga routines and is called the pose of the child.

3. When doing this exercise it is important that both your shoulders remain on the floor. Lie on your back with your arms resting beside your body. Slowly draw your knees in to your chest and to the count of four lower both knees down to the floor on your right side. Rest there for two seconds, then again to the count of four, return your knees to your chest. Repeat on the other side.

How many should you do? Since these exercises are a form of relief for backache they can be done regularly – say twice or three times each day. Three or four repetitions of 1 and 3 will be enough at each session, whilst position 2 can be held for as long as is comfortable.

This tones the waist and stretches the spine.

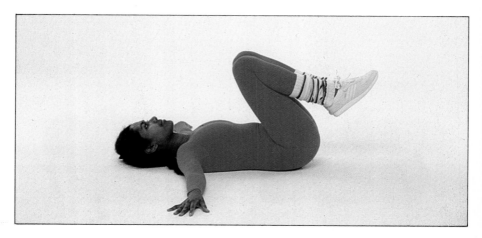

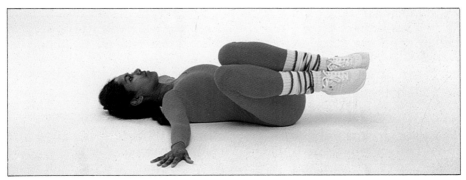

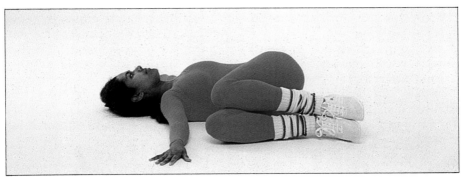

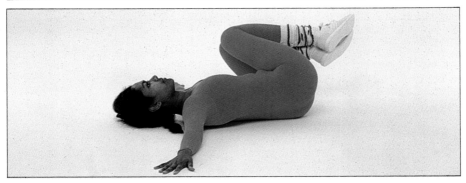

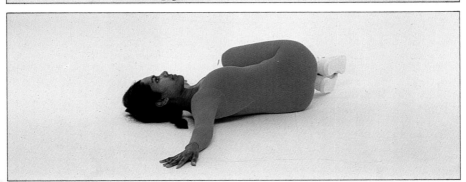

Ribs and waist

Waist exercises are often a cause of lower backache when people begin exercising. So for these exercises make sure that you are standing correctly so as not to put strain on your back: keep most of your weight on the front of your feet and be careful not to lean backwards; don't push your hips forward when leaning over to the side.

Suppleness and toning – ribs

These are referred to by teachers as isolation exercises. It is a good idea to watch yourself in a mirror. First, standing with feet a little apart, and your hands placed on your ribcage, breathe in gently and feel your lungs expand. Exhale gently; repeat three or four times.

Now for the isolation movement. With your hands either by your sides or holding your ribcage, lift your ribcage high out of your waist. Now, gently ease your ribcage over to the left of your body, and then slowly over to the right. Don't move your hips.

Don't overdo this one.

When you have mastered this movement you can progress to the forward and backwards ribcage stretch. For this, extend your ribcage forward in front of you, and slowly contract as though someone has kicked you in the ribs. Strange feeling, isn't it?

Check in a mirror that you're starting with the correct posture (*right*).

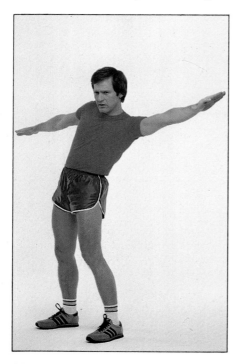
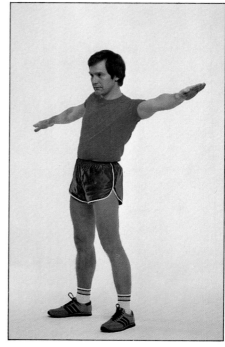

58

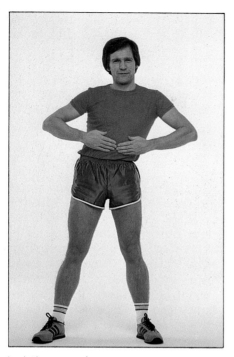
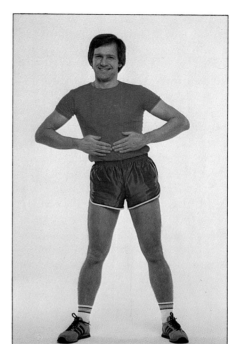

Isolation exercises

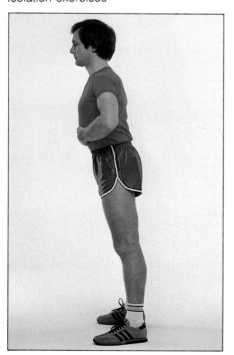
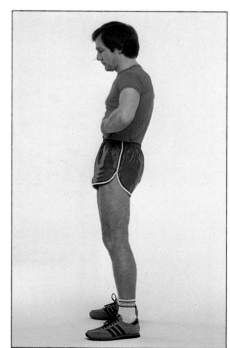

If you think that you have managed these fairly well, why not try the hardest of them all? Circle the ribs around to the right, and then make a full circle to the left.

How many should you do?   Two repetitions in each direction for all these exercises is enough.

Suppleness and toning – waist

This exercise is commonly demonstrated in keep-fit groups and in exercise manuals, yet rarely have I seen a warning against using the spine instead of the waist.

Stand with feet apart and arms by your sides; shoulders relaxed and head up, and don't forget to keep most of your weight on the front of your feet. Now lean over to your left-hand side, lowering your left hand down the side of your leg and letting your right arm slide up to allow maximum movement. In order to do this correctly, let your head fall on to your shoulder and be extremely careful not to let your hips come forward. Don't try to touch your ankle as so many people do, but gently ease your body down to the side, eight times on each side. One further point: when reaching down your leg, don't let your hips swing out to

Ribcage circling

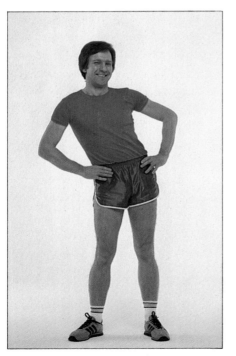
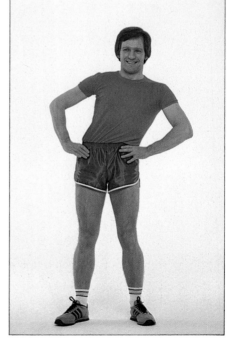

Touching your ankle (*right*) may look harder but won't give you the same stretch at the waist (*below*) and could cause backache.

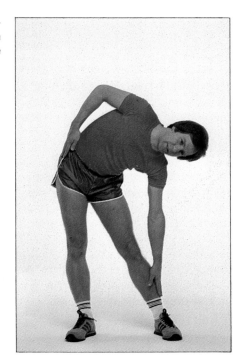

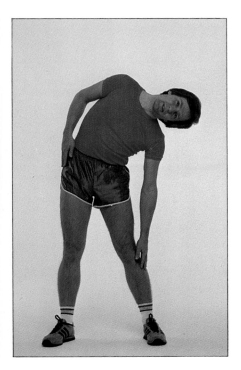

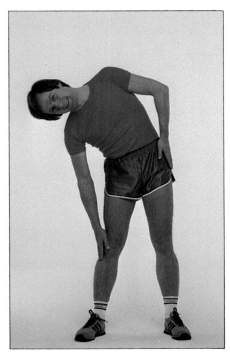

the opposite side. Although this hip movement will enable you to reach further down it will be putting more strain on your spine instead of stretching the waist.

How many should you do? Beginners, repeat eight stretches each side daily; fairly fit, eight on each side up to three repetitions; even fitter, begin as for fairly fit and increase gradually to six repetitions.

Waist shaper

This exercise is undoubtedly a tough one and should only be attempted by those who feel fairly fit and supple. At the first sign of backache, do slow down or stop and have a rest.

Stand with feet a little apart and arms at shoulder level stretched out to your sides. Pull your tummy in and remember, weight off your heels! Now gently stretch over to the left. Hold that stretch for two seconds and slowly pull your right arm over your head so that both arms are in line with your side. You must tilt your head on to your shoulder so that you can really pull your arm well over. Now bend your knees a little and straighten them, and again, bend your knees and straighten them, and gently relax both arms down in front of you and roll up to a standing

The waist shaper

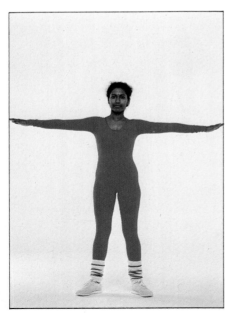 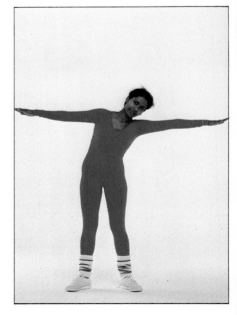

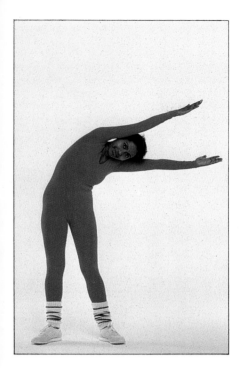

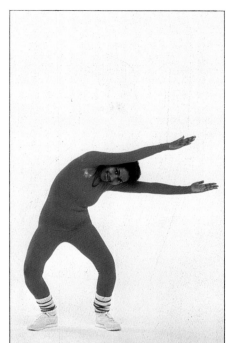

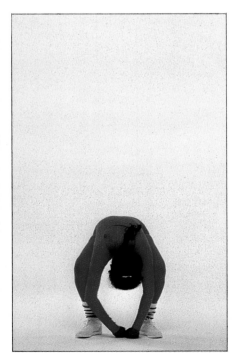

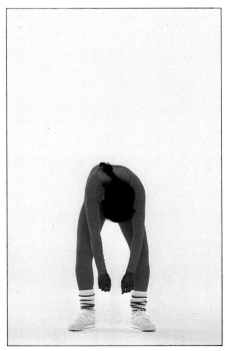

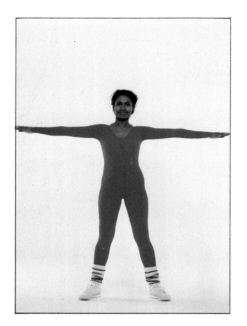

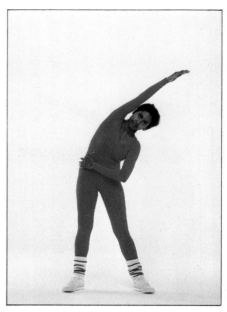

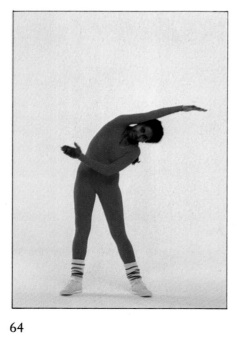

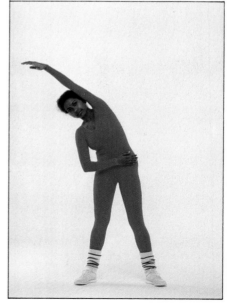

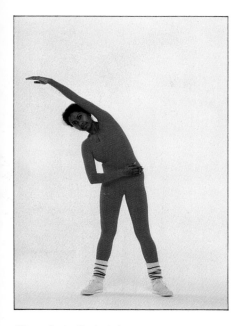
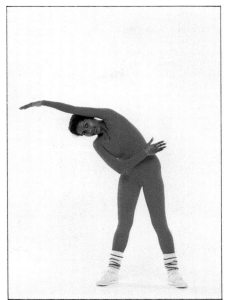

The windmill stretch

position, ready to begin the sequence again on the other side. Repeat twice on each side, building gradually up to six repetitions.

The windmill stretch
A gentle yet effective exercise that can be done just before you go to bed or when you get up, rather than during your workout.

Standing with feet apart, lift your right arm over your head and lean to the left, meanwhile letting your left arm cradle to the right as though you were holding a baby in it. Now gently, push your left arm and pull with your right arm. This pushing and pulling motion should be very smooth and gentle and you should feel quite a pull on the waist. As always, repeat the exercise on the other side.

How many should you do?   All abilities: begin with just four pulls and build up to twelve as and when you feel ready.

Jogging
This section applies only to those who consider themselves reasonably fit and who are under forty-five. Anyone over 20 lb (10 kg) overweight

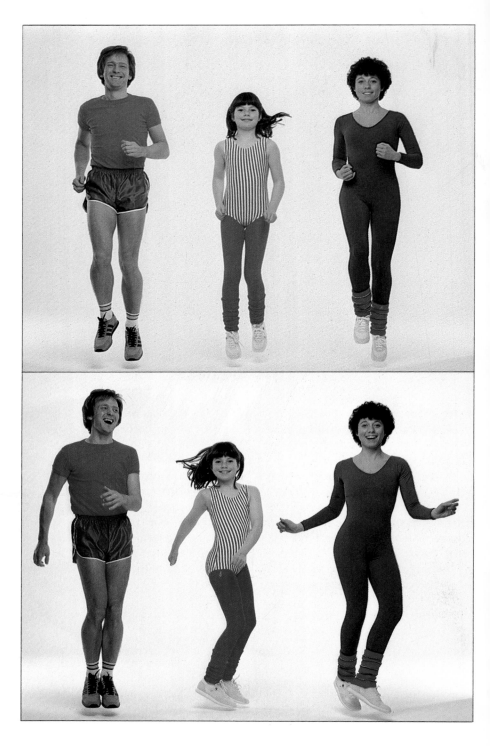

Different styles of aerobic jogging: running, *above*, twisting, *below*

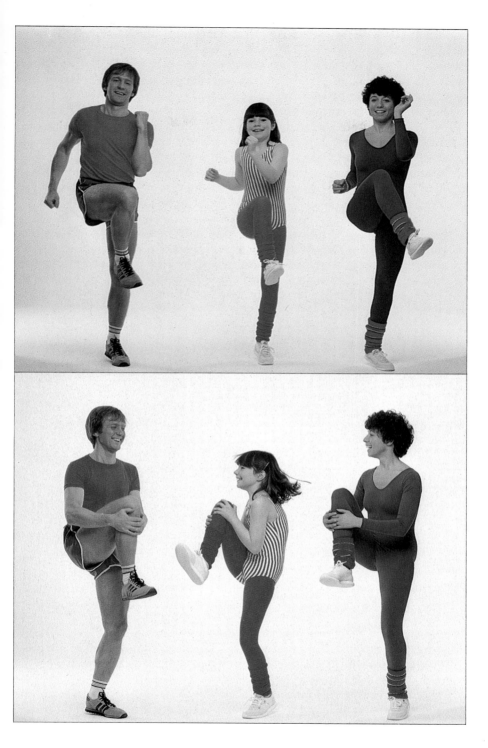

Touching the opposite elbow to the knee, *above*, and knee hugging, *below*

should check with his or her doctor before doing these exercises (see the weight chart in Chapter 1). If you are just over the normal weight and cannot see any reason why not to, have a go, but very gently to begin with. At the first sign of pain, cramp, dizziness, sickness or feeling faint, slow down to a stop, and rest or get aid.

Warning: These exercises are described as aerobic as they increase the entry of air (oxygen) into the body. They are likely to burn up your sugars quickly so test before and after once or twice when you begin to practise them, to see roughly how much energy you use up.

Don't forget either that after you have stopped jogging your body is still keyed up and will continue to burn energy at a slightly faster rate than normal. It is hard to be specific about how long this post-exercise period lasts for any one person, but you should be aware of it and keep a check after your workout for the first few times. I use this type of exercise if ever I discover that my sugar is a little too high and I want to bring it down just before I go to bed. I find that five to ten minutes of this jogging will bring my blood sugar down from say 11 to 7 mmol per litre (200 to 150 mg per 100 ml), which is just about right for going to bed.

If possible choose a piece of music to do the exercises to as that will keep you going. Remember that jogging is running on the spot at regular speed. Begin very gently and try to land without too much strain on your feet. Keep your hands relaxed and aim to keep your ankles down as you land. This will help prevent straining. Vary the routine of jogging, skipping or twisting and the time will go quickly. You can also vary the number of times you do a movement, for example, starting with eight, then four, then two, then one; back to two, four and eight again.

How much should you do? Beginners, no more than two minutes; fairly fit, two to six minutes (building up slowly); even fitter, up to twelve minutes.

Twelve minutes may not seem a very long time but I can tell you it will when you are jogging and twisting!

Hips and buttocks

Without doubt, it is the hips and buttocks that take the prize for the most moans, especially among women. The following exercises are great for strengthening the legs, tummy and hips and also for firming up the buttocks as you get trim.

There are two positions for this group, standing and lying on the floor. Don't think that the lying on the floor ones are going to be easier! Try some standing exercises first.

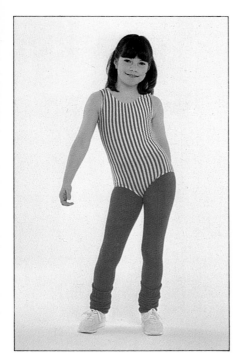

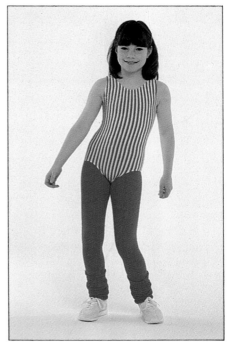

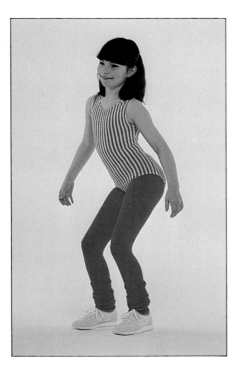

Hip swivels

With feet a little apart, knees slightly bent and hands on your hips, squeeze your bottom muscles just a little and circle your hips in a tight circle, first to the left then to the right. After a couple of swivels in each direction, swing your hips forwards and backwards. (This exercise is often used for pregnancy preparation and for post-natal exercises.)

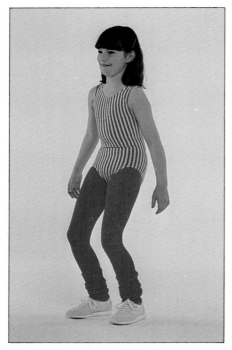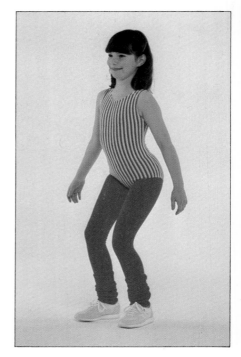

The pelvic tilt

Pelvic tilt

Now, again with knees a little bent, and feet slightly apart, hands out in front for balance, squeeze your bottom muscles and tilt your pelvic muscles forwards, then gently tilt back so that your bottom is sticking out.

How many should you do? Repeat the first set four times, building up to eight. Do the second eight times. But don't do these exercises too frantically or you may get a lower backache.

The big squeeze

This exercise always brings a big smile to my students' faces, but it certainly gets those flabby muscles working.

With feet apart, hands relaxed by your sides and knees slightly bent, squeeze your bottom for the count of five seconds and then gently release the tension. Repeat six times. By the way, don't forget to smile!

Floor exercises for buttocks and hips

Lie down on the floor, relax your spine and bend your knees so that both feet are flat on the floor and your heels are close to your thighs. With arms resting by your sides, you are ready to begin.

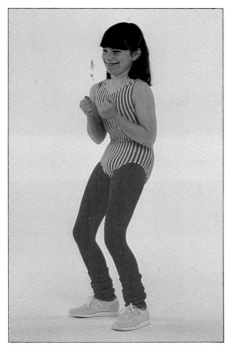 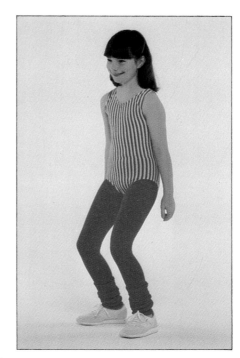

You're never too old to start this exercise!

This is the basic floor position; notice how the fingertips are nearly touching the heels.

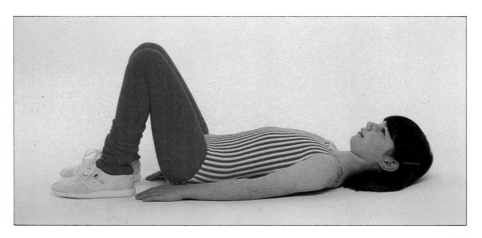

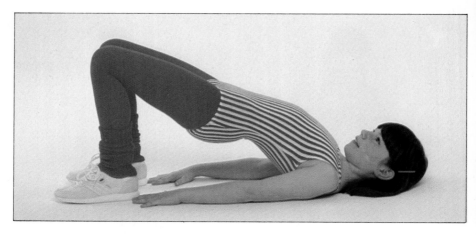

The raised basic position

Gently raise your spine off the floor so that you are taking most of your weight on your shoulders and feet. From this starting position there are three variations. In between each sequence slowly lower your back to the floor and curl your knees up to your chest, giving them a hug with your arms for a couple of seconds before returning to the starting position again. This will prevent back or abdominal muscle strain.

1. From the starting position, gently squeeze your bottom muscles and hold for one second, then release the squeeze. Don't let your bottom lower towards the floor. You will notice that your hips rise with each squeeze. Begin by doing just six and build up gradually to thirty times over several weeks.

The full squeeze

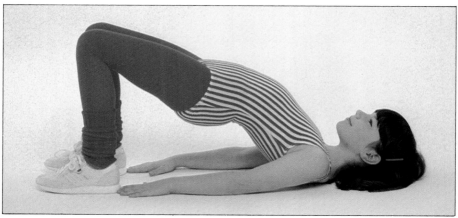

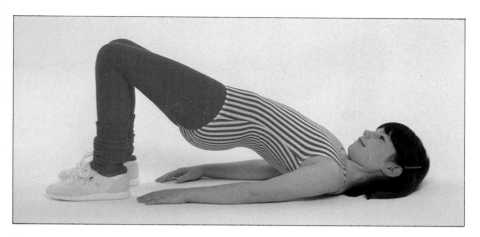

The left squeeze, *top*, the right squeeze, *middle*, and knee touching, *below*

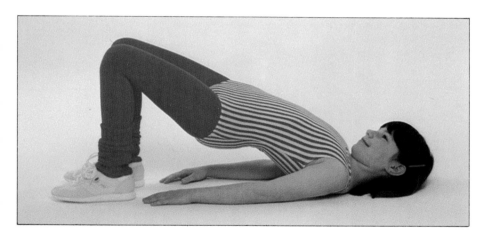

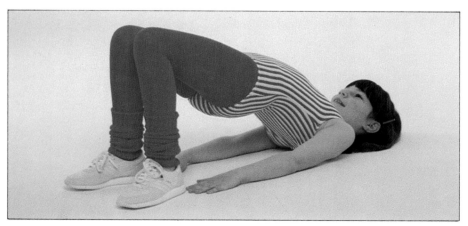

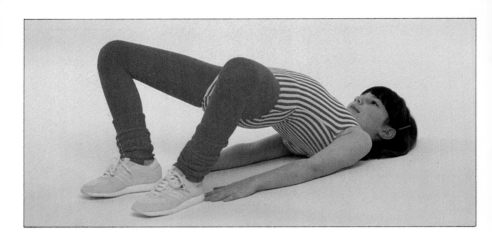

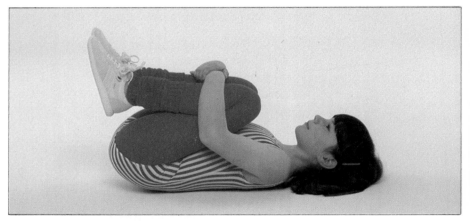

(*Top*) Knees apart, the final position in exercise 3.

When you are doing any of these exercises, at the first sign of lower back strain take up the relaxed position (*above*) and wait for another time to try again.

2. From the starting position, squeeze your left buttock only and then squeeze only the right one. Don't lower your hips in between squeezes. Begin by doing six repetitions and build up to thirty gradually, as in 1.

3. This part of the exercise really firms up the inside of your thighs. From the starting position, gently bring your knees together until they touch each other and then let them fall apart. So, together and apart, together and apart. Begin with just four of these and build up to twelve. This is quite a tough one, so don't overdo it!

The bouncer

One last quick and easy exercise which can be done almost anywhere . . .
It not only firms up your backside, but also the backs of your legs, from
the ankles to the tops of your thighs.

Stand with feet together, hands relaxed by your sides, and keeping
your legs straight, raise both heels off the floor. Lower. Repeat fairly
quickly, starting with about twenty and building up to fifty.

Legs

No routine is complete without exercises for the thighs and legs. Again,
the overweight will benefit from these since they will tone up muscle as
you lose weight – but leg exercises are always popular with everybody,
and they certainly improve the shape rapidly if they are done regularly.
Each one tones a different part, so try not to leave any out.

The bouncer: notice that the heels barely touch the floor before you rise up to the ball
of the feet again. The faster you bounce the tougher it becomes.

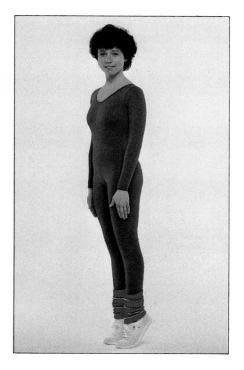 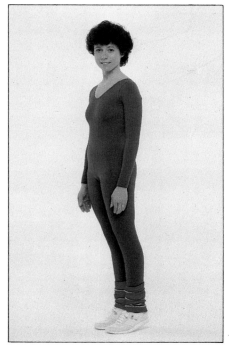

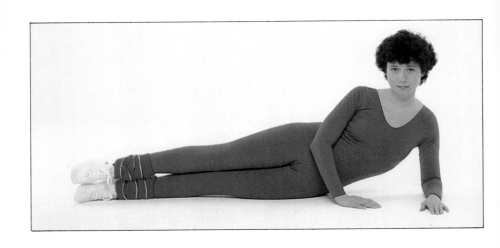

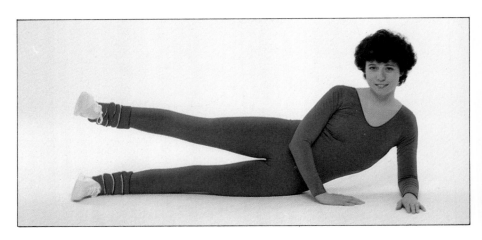

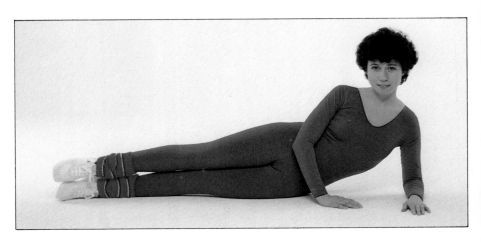

1. Lie on your side with one leg resting on top of the other. Support yourself on your elbow (protect your bony elbow with a towel if necessary). Now lift and lower the top leg rhythmically about 12 to 18 in (30 to 45 cms), alternating between pointed and flexed foot. Then relax your leg by bending your knee into your tummy and gently stretching it out four times.

    Begin with eight repetitions on each side and build up to thirty-two over a period of a month or so.

Leg lifts: aim to stretch the leg from the hip to the foot to get the full benefit.

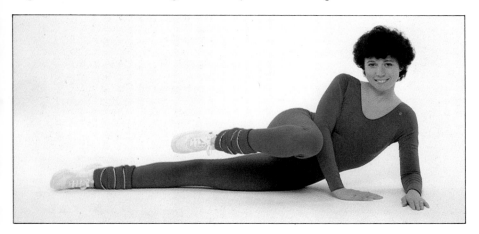

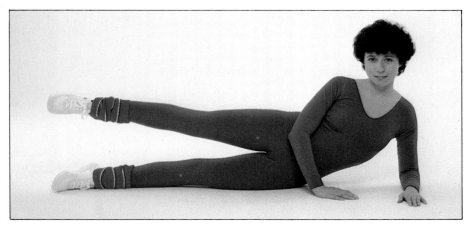

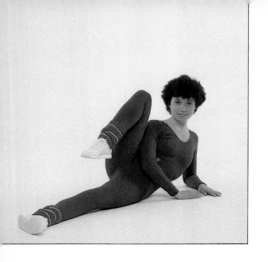
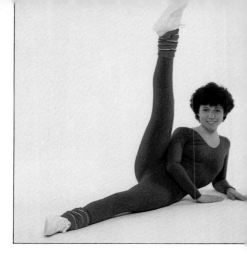
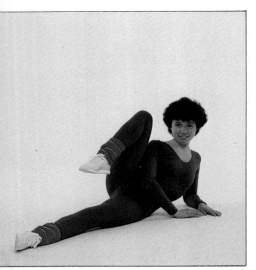
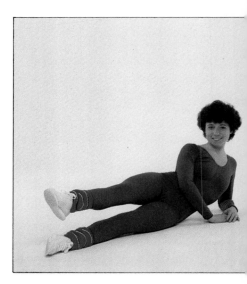

The toe to thigh toner: when doing this exercise don't let your body roll backwards but try to remain up on your hips.

2. Now, raise the leg and stretch it up with toes pointed rather than flexed, bend down and stretch out four times, then repeat four times with the foot flexed. Don't worry if you can't straighten your leg completely. This exercise is quite tough on the backs of your legs and more flexibility will come with practice. Always do the same number of repetitions on the other side.

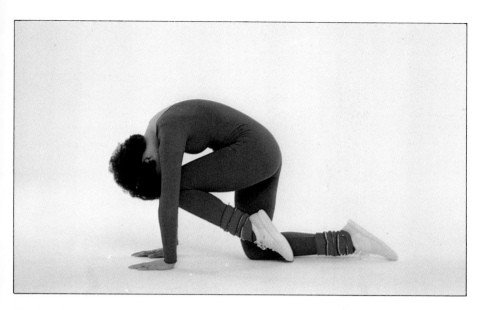

The leg thrust

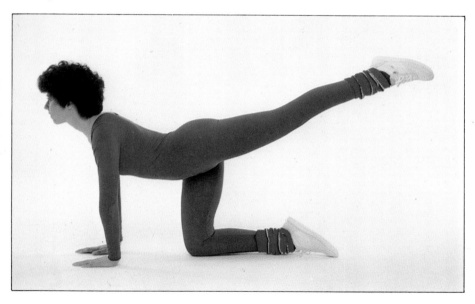

3. Turning on to all fours, bend your right knee in to your chest and lower your head to touch it and then stretch out your leg behind you and stretch your head up. Bend your knee in again. Repeat this exercise four times on each leg to begin with and build up to twelve.

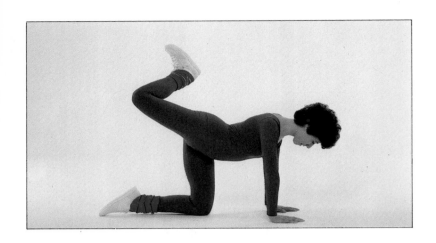

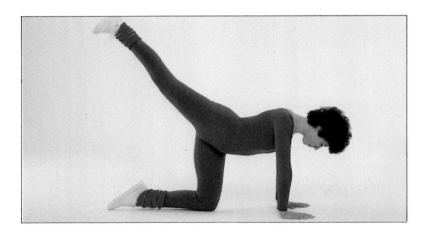

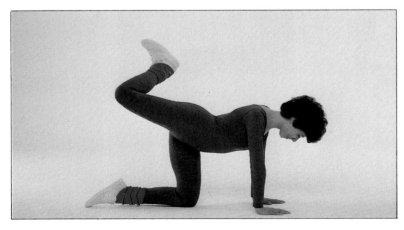

The donkey kick

Donkey kick

This exercise is a favourite with most of my students since it really stretches the legs and tones up lumpy thighs and buttocks.

On all fours, bend your right leg, keeping your foot flexed, and push the leg up and back, with foot flexed all the time.

How many should you do? Start with four and build up to twelve kicks with each leg.

Thigh tone-up

Sit on the floor with legs wide apart and arms in front of you. Lower your spine and breathe out, then raise your spine out of your hips and breathe in. Continue breathing gently and stay in the raised position, bending both knees a little. Don't move your heels but flex your toes. Now lower your knees to the floor and point your toes.

How many should you do? Bend, flex, stretch and point eight times to begin with and gradually build up to twenty.

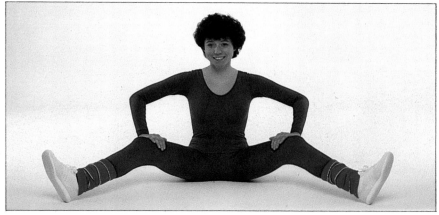

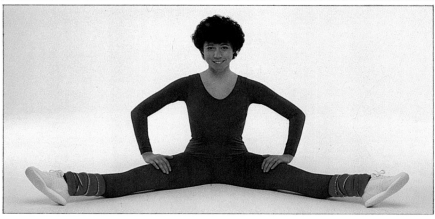

The thigh tone-up

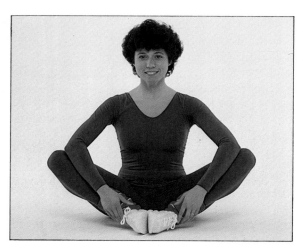

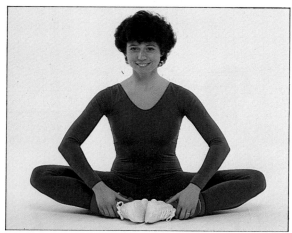

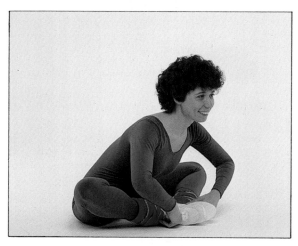

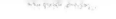

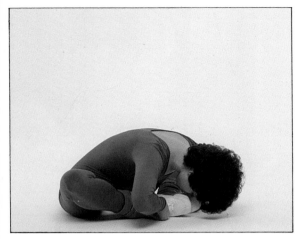

The inner thigh stretch: these exercises done regularly will help to improve the strength and suppleness of the lower spine as well as tone the inner thighs.

Inner thigh stretch
Bring your feet as close together as possible and hold on to your ankles, feeling the stretch of muscles at the inside top of your thighs. Gently bounce your knees to loosen up and stretch the inner thigh muscles. When relaxed, bend forward and with a flat back and shoulders down, gently bounce forward to four counts, then do four bounces trying to place your forehead on your toes at each bounce.

How many should you do?   Begin with four repetitions, building up gradually to as many as you like.

Toning the abdomen

You do not have to be overweight to have a saggy abdomen. We tend to assess our size by the pouch sitting in front of us and if you recognize yourself as pouchy you may need to lose some weight. For a lot of people, however, especially new mothers or people who lead very sedentary lives, these muscles simply need gentle and regular toning. A few minutes each day makes an enormous difference to the figure and posture.

Abdomen exercises should never be done immediately after a heavy snack. If you are insulin-dependent, though, do check your sugar first and make sure that you have enough to keep you going as these burn up energy rather quickly.

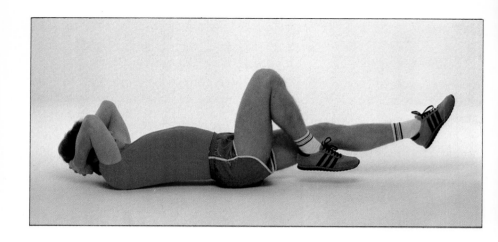

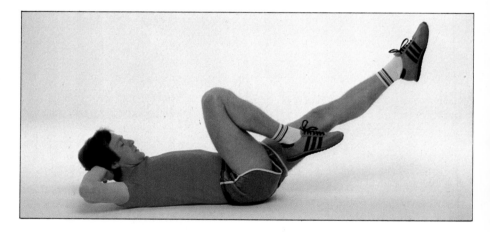

Note how the spine arches off the floor in the incorrect position (*top*). The lower picture shows the correct position and is the start of the full sequence.

Among the abdomen exercises devised for the recent keep-fit boom, some are unnecessarily strenuous, and possibly harmful. Since the idea is to improve your health and stamina gradually, I include just a couple of basic exercises that are quite safe for people of all ages and abilities.

It is absolutely essential to start from the correct position or you will suffer from backache! Always keep your back flat on the floor.

Take up the correct floor position and clasp your hands behind your head so that your elbows are stretched out sideways. Bring your knees slowly in towards your chest.

84

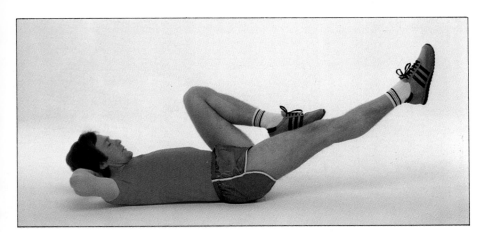

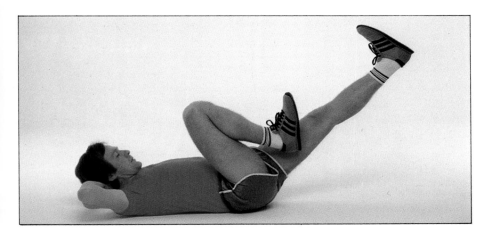

The *top picture* shows the pointing sequence, and the *lower* the beginning of the flexing.

In your own time, stretch out each leg alternately, as in the second photograph, *not* as in the first. If you try to stretch your legs out close to floor level, your spine will probably arch to maintain control and you will no longer be using your abdomen muscles but straining your spine.

Finish with your knees resting on your chest.

1. Now you have mastered the correct floor position, begin the full sequence: stretch your legs out alternately and point your toes, left, right, left, right.

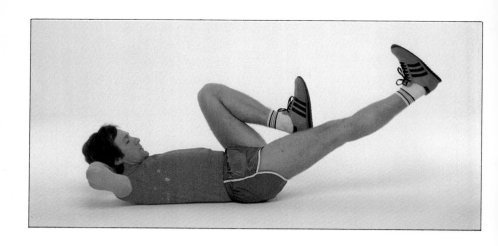

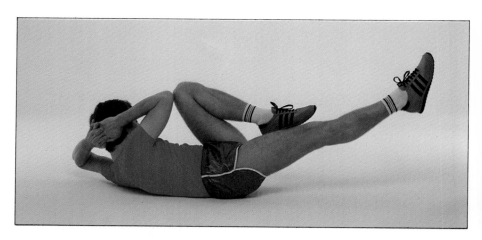

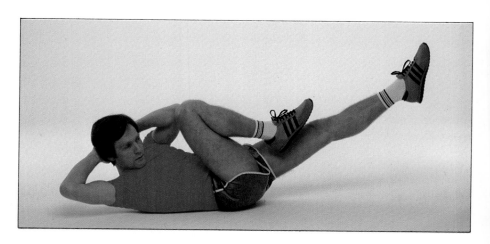

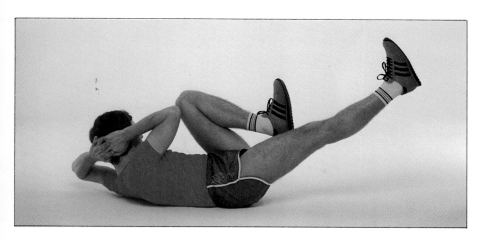

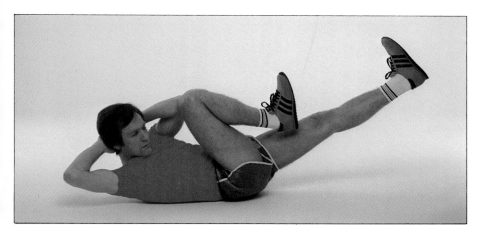

Try not to rush the sequence — feel the full extent of the stretch on each leg.

Next, with your feet flexed continue stretching your legs out, left, right, left, right. Bring your knees back to your chest. Relax for a few seconds. Now point your toes again, and this time bring your right elbow up to touch your left knee and then change so that your left elbow touches your right knee.

Do this four times with pointed toes, then repeat four times with flexed toes.

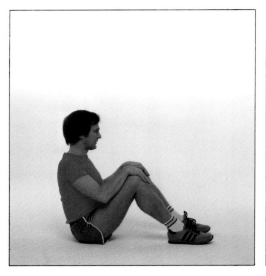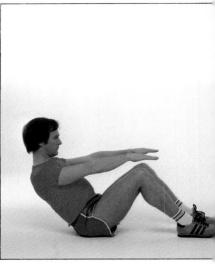

The abdomen toner: this is one of the more advanced exercises.

It is important to keep a straight spine all the time so as not to cause lower backache.

2. Sit with your knees bent up and your feet on the floor, hip distance apart. Put your hands on your knees. Relax from the top of your spine – now slowly sit up with a good straight spine and hold the position for the count of five.

   Next, leave hold of your knees and lean back so that with outstretched arms your hands are just hovering over your kneecaps. Slowly raise your left hand so that your elbow rests just by your ear and then lower your arm again and do the same with your right arm. Repeat four times, then pull up to the sitting position with a rope-tugging movement.

How many should you do? Repeat this alternating lifting and lowering four times to begin with and build up to twelve.

If you can master these few exercises adequately, there shouldn't be any need to try other variations other than for the fun of it, but just one more word of warning: some exercise manuals encourage speedy sit-ups and exercises with legs outstretched just a few centimetres from the floor to build up stomach muscle stamina. If done unsupervised or by the not-so-strong these strain your spine. Remember, the idea of the exercises is to improve your health and well-being not to leave you with crippling aches and pains.

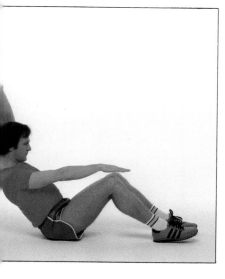
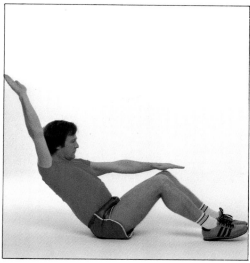
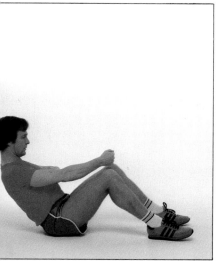
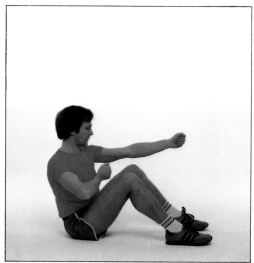

The cool-down

It is as important to slow down gently from an exercise routine as to start with the warm-up exercises. Ending with your pulse racing and in a state of excitement will cause unnecessarily fast burning of your sugars for too long afterwards. Apart from this danger to your diabetes, there is the effect on your muscles and joints. Stopping suddenly when your

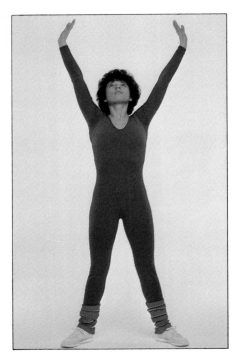
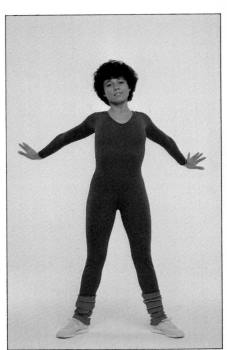
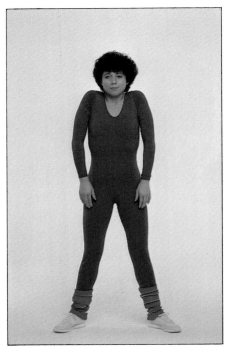
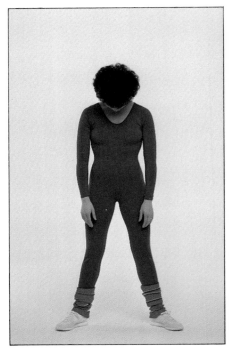

muscles are hot may lead to seizing up and cramps. Even top athletic sportsmen continue to run at a slower pace after they have passed the finishing line to slow their heartbeat rates down.

In my classes I finish with at least thirty seconds of relaxation (see page 16), allowing everyone to choose his or her most comfortable position, be it lying down or standing up, followed by a few final stretches. As for the warm-up, these are done in a standing position with the correct posture:

1. Gently lift your arms up above your head to the count of four and exhale. Then lower your arms to the count of four.
2. Raise your arms up in front of you to the count of four and gently circle them behind you.
3. Finally do a couple of shoulder shrugs before flopping to a limp, totally relaxed position.

The cool down: *top left*, arm raising; *top right*, full arm circling; *bottom left*, shoulder shrug; *bottom right*, complete flop

5 SPECIAL ROUTINES

In this chapter, I give a series of exercise routines for special conditions – for people who do not have time to do the whole workout in Chapter 4, and for those who should stick to the gentler exercises. I use exercises that are part of the full workout, so you will still be getting the maximum benefit if you keep doing them regularly to the best of your ability.

A shortened workout

Setting aside thirty minutes or more every day is often too much to keep up for long; there are bound to be days when you are too rushed to think about your exercise routine. There are two ways of coping with exercise on these hectic days:

1. Include some of my exercise ideas, like walking upstairs, ankle circling (page 51) while you are on your way to work, or in the work place. Do a few shoulder shrugs and neck rolls (pages 43–4) in your lunch hour and walk briskly and as much as you can during that day.

2. Better still, allow just five minutes for exercise in the morning and maybe five more minutes before you go to bed.

Include:
- a warm-up stretch or two (Achilles tendon and monkey swings, pages 36, 41)
- a few circulation exercises (ankle or arm circles, pages 48, 50)
- one to ease the spine (ripple, page 53)
- a hip swivel (page 69)
- one leg toner (page 76)
- one abdomen exercise (page 84)
- one minute's relaxation pose (page 55).

Pregnancy

It is important to keep fit during pregnancy, but as the months progress you will have to reduce the vigour of your exercise routine. The first

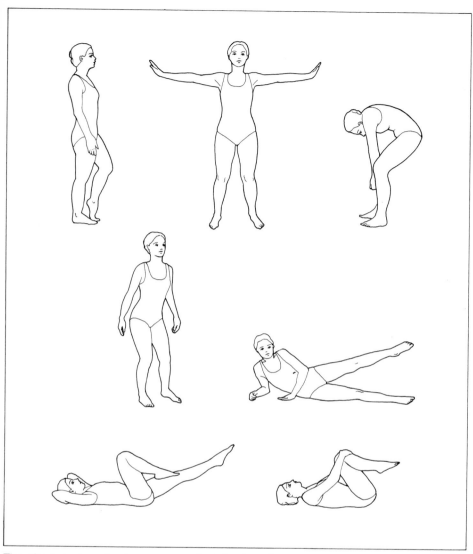

The shortened workout: you can adjust the length according to the amount of time you have to spare.

sequence I give is for the first three months, the later one for the third to the sixth, or until the bulge makes it uncomfortable to exercise.

1. Following the warm-up (page 36), do the big stretch to get the blood circulating and to help you feel alert: stand with feet apart and raise your arms above your head, keeping the shoulders relaxed. Hold for five, gently breathe out and lower your arms.

2. Head, neck and shoulder tension: follow the exercises on page 42.

3. The spine: during pregnancy your spine will be asked to work overtime so it is wise to spend a few minutes each day helping it become strong and supple. Try the exercises on page 53.

4. Hips and pelvic muscles: during a natural birth, the pelvic muscles are stretched, so it is a good idea to start strengthening the lower part of your body from the beginning of the pregnancy. Don't overdo these exercises and remember to build up gradually (see page 68).

5. Legs and feet: the extra weight in pregnancy will cause aching legs and tired feet. Being diabetic may mean too that your general circulation isn't as good as it should be. Pay even more attention to your legs and feet from now on and start some of the exercises on page 75 on a regular basis.

From the third to the sixth month the bulge starts showing. If during this period your diabetes and general health are in good order, regular exercise including plenty of walking and swimming will be most beneficial.

Assuming your doctor has not advised against it, you may like to try some relaxing and suppling exercises at home. As always, aim to build up gradually. Most positions should be held for a count of five but as you improve you may be able to hold some of them for up to fifteen seconds.

First, always practise the warm-up stretches, with emphasis on stretching out the muscles at the back of the foot, heel and leg (see page 37). If these muscles are not warmed up you may easily pull them and cause unnecessary injury.

Following the warm-up, try the following poses – for the first week just concentrate on a couple of poses each day.

The tailor pose
Sit on the floor (not the bed as it is too soft), in a cross-legged position. Place your hands on your knees, relax your shoulders and neck. Allow the spine to relax and drop back on to the hips. Gently breathe in and pull the spine back out of the hips so that it is once again tall and erect. Hold the tall position for five seconds and gently breathe out again, allowing the spine to relax completely.

Uncurl your legs and shake them out to keep the blood flowing and prevent cramp.

The squat
Many women find the squatting position natural and comfortable during

94

Top and middle: the tailor pose

Bottom: the squat

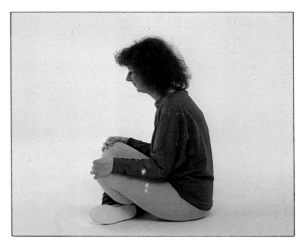

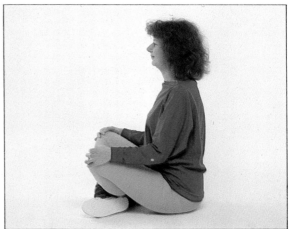

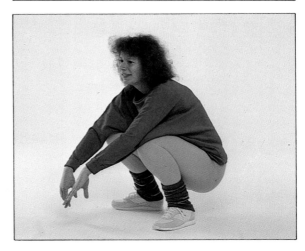

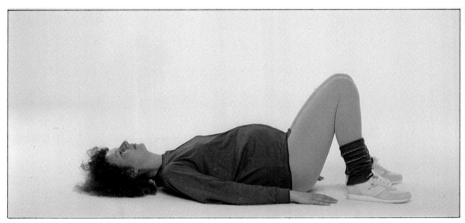

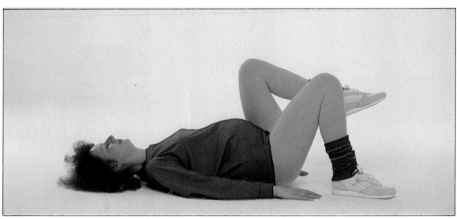

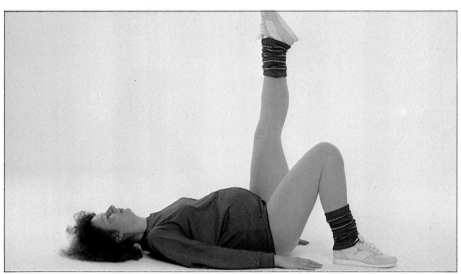

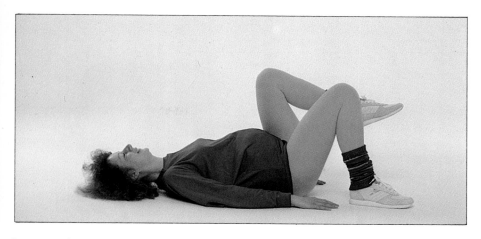

Leg stretches: naturally, the larger you are the harder it will be to extend your leg fully, so just do the best you can. Try to keep your shoulders and neck relaxed on to the floor throughout the sequence.

childbirth and it is a good idea to become familiar with it early on. Practise the position for as long as is comfortable.

Leg stretches

Lie flat on the floor with your arms by your sides; don't use a cushion for support but try to let your spine relax flat into the floor so that you cannot move your hands below the hollow of the spine. This will prevent the possibility of lower backache (see illustration on page 84). First bend your knees up with your feet firmly on the floor. Bend one knee into your chest, then raise the leg, stretching towards the ceiling. Bend and stretch four times, then repeat with the other leg.

Repeated regularly, this exercise builds up strength in the legs which will help to carry the extra weight. By keeping your legs higher than your head for a couple of minutes each day you are also encouraging better overall circulation and releasing tension.

How many should you do?   Begin with four and build up to twelve.

The cat

This is a useful aid to relaxation, relieving any tension in the lower spine, and it can be done as often as you like.

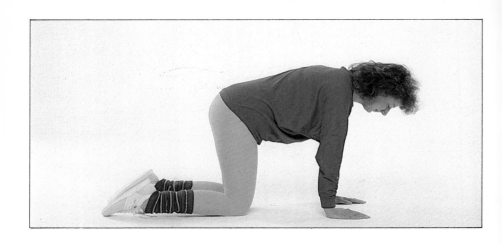

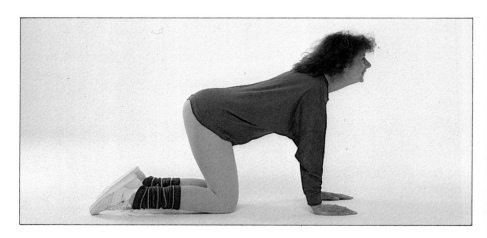

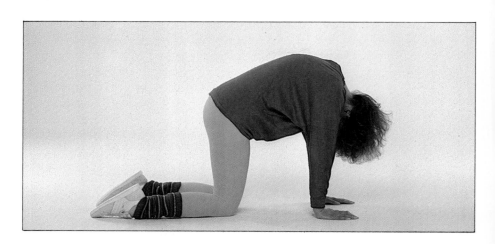

Starting on all fours, inhale slowly to the count of four, hollowing your spine, then exhale, raising your spine and letting your head and neck relax completely.

Relaxation phase

It is never too soon to learn to relax, whether or not you are pregnant. Here is one pose to aid relaxation (see also page 16).

Lie on the floor with your legs resting on a small piece of soft furniture or on a few cushions, so that your feet are above your head. Some people prefer to relax in total or semi-darkness, whilst others enjoy full daylight. It doesn't matter which you choose. Let your arms and hands rest calmly by your sides with the palms of your hands upwards and feel your head, neck and shoulders relax into the floor, allowing your eyes to close lightly. Rest in this position for as long as it's comfortable.

Special problems

Following the lessons learnt from medical research, the proportion of diabetics who suffer acute upsets is decreasing, and the proportion suffering more chronic problems should also decrease. Nowadays, the new diabetic is stabilized rapidly, and if on insulin is taught how to test his or her own blood sugars right from the start, and because of this the majority of diabetics should lead healthy and long lives like non-diabetics. For a few, however, complications like eyesight problems and

Left, the cat, and *below*, the relaxation pose. Try to relax for at least a few minutes each day, not too soon after a main meal.

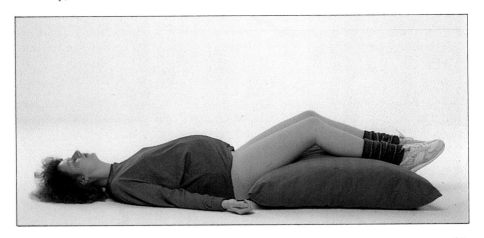

loss of sensation in the extremities may be inevitable. There is also a percentage of diabetics who are wheelchair-bound, not because of their diabetes but for some other reason.

What about exercise? Undoubtedly, loss of sight, limb or mobility makes it difficult. Yet daily movement is tremendously helpful, especially for circulation and maintaining strength in the mobile limbs, and in the long run enjoyable. Here I suggest a routine for the disabled or chair-bound that can be done anywhere.

Loss of balance and confidence may mean that greater effort is needed to start but there are several exercises in this book that can be done. Read through Chapter 4 to see for yourself which exercises you think you will be able to try (those marked with an asterisk are probably the most suitable). What is right for you, may not be right for the next person.

For the partially sighted Make sure that someone is around when you first exercise, just in case of any difficulties. Do all standing up exercises holding on to something to help you balance – for example, the back of a sturdy chair.

For the less mobile Many of the exercises can be adapted so that you can do them from a chair or even a bed (again note the ones marked with an asterisk), but don't try any for the first time when you are alone, unless you are quite confident of your physical abilities.

- Whatever your problem, always try to include a warm-up exercise, a few circulation exercises and a relaxation stretch (see pages 37, 46, 41).
- The bed-bound person may manage to do the fist clenching, piano playing and toe and foot circulation exercises (see pages 46, 50).
- A partially mobile person might try some of the hip, leg or abdomen exercises (see pages 68, 75, 83). Begin with the minimum of repetitions though.

Here are a few more you can choose from. When you try these exercises, don't force stiff joints or try any movement that you find awkward or painful. It may take a little time before you can do them all.

Waist mobility Sit up straight on an upright chair, then gently twist your upper body to the right so that you are looking over your right shoulder. Hold that twist for the count of three and then slowly return to the front. Repeat on the left side.

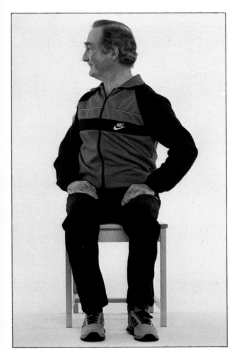
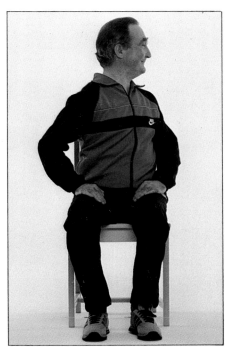

Waist mobility: when doing these exercises make sure that your feet are resting firmly on the floor and they do not move while you turn.

Feet   Sitting on an upright chair, cross one leg over the other if you can. If you find this difficult, just lift your foot off the floor a few inches. Starting with the right foot, gently circle your ankle three times to the right and then back three times to the left. Repeat the exercise with the other foot.

Head, shoulders, neck   (See illustration page 43)
1. Sitting on your chair, just let your head fall forward, then gently lift it up. Drop your right ear down towards your right shoulder – without lifting your shoulder towards your ear. Do the same with the left ear.
2. Bring both shoulders up towards your ear lobes, hold for three seconds and then let them drop and relax.

How many should you do?   Start with two repetitions of each exercise that you can do and increase to four. You can build up very gradually to sixteen or more so long as you suffer no discomfort.

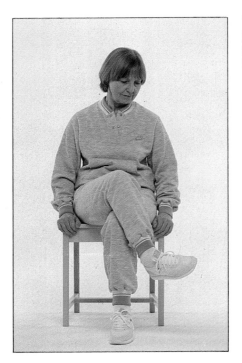

This is a particularly good exercise to do just before going to bed and first thing in the morning since it increases the blood flow to the coldest part of the body.

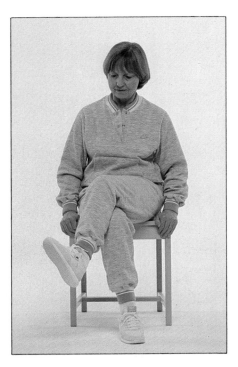

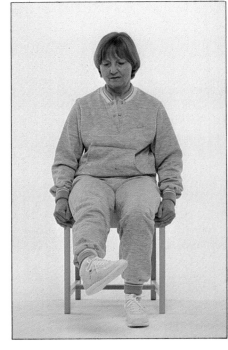

You may find that your local association for the disabled or the blind holds regular social and exercise sessions, and this is certainly a pleasant way to do exercise. Remember if you join, though, to mention your diabetes and to keep yourself prepared with sufficient carbohydrate foods just in case of hypos. Perhaps you are even more ambitious and want to join in, say, wheelchair sports. In the UK the Disabled Living Foundation are well aware of the need to bring exercise and sports to disabled people, and there are now sporting events and Olympic games for disabled groups worldwide.

USEFUL ADDRESSES

UNITED KINGDOM

Action on Smoking and Health (ASH)
5-11 Mortimer Street
London W1N 7RH

Age Concern (Head London Office)
Bernard Sunley House
60 Pitcairn Road
Mitcham
Surrey CR4 3LL

The British Diabetic Association Ltd
10 Queen Anne Street
London W1

British Sports Association for the Disabled
Hayward House
Barnard Crescent
Aylesbury
Bucks HB21 8PP

The Disabled Living Foundation
346 Kensington High Street
London W14 8NS

Health Education Council
78 New Oxford Street
London WC1A 1AH

Keep Fit Association
16 Upper Woburn Place
London WC1H 0QG

Ramblers Association
1-5 Wandsworth Road
London SW8 2LJ

The Sports Council
PO Box 480
Jubilee Stand
Crystal Palace National
Sports Centre
Ledrington Road
London SE19 2BQ

UNITED STATES

The American Diabetes Association
2 Park Avenue
New York, NY 10016

Juvenile Diabetes Foundation
60 Madison Avenue
New York, NY 10010

National Diabetes Information Clearing House
Box NDIC
Bethesda, MD 20205

CANADA

The Canadian Diabetes Association
(National Office)
78 Bond Street
Toronto
Ontario M5B 2J8

AUSTRALIA

Doctors and other professionals in the field of diabetes should contact:
The Australian Diabetic Society
c/o Endocrine Unit
St Vincent's Hospital
Fitzroy
Victoria 3065

Australian Diabetes Foundation
27 Brewer Street
East Perth
W.A. 6000

Diabetes Youth Foundation of Australia
36 Spring Street
Bondi Junction
NSW 2022

Diabetes Association of the A.C.T.
Woden Valley Hospital
Garren A.C.T. 2606
Tel: (062) 83 2139

Diabetes Foundation of Victoria
100 Collins Street
Melbourne VIC. 3000
Tel: (03) 63 8793

Diabetic Association of NSW
250 Pitt Street
Sydney NSW 2000
Tel: (02) 264 6851

Diabetic Association of Queensland
Room 122 Canberra Hotel
Ann Street
Brisbane QLD 4000
Tel: (07) 229 1986

Diabetic Association of Western Australia
19 Irwin Street
Perth W.A. 6000
Tel: (09) 325 7174

Tasmanian Diabetic Association, Inc.
86 Hampden Road
Bay Point
Hobart TAS. 7000
Tel: (002) 34 5223

Diabetic Association of S.A. Inc.
Eleanor Harrold Building
Frome Road
Adelaide S.A. 5000
Tel: (08) 223 7848

NEW ZEALAND

The New Zealand Diabetic Association
PO Box 3656
Wellington

SOUTH AFRICA

The South African Diabetic Association
PO Box 10998
Johannesburg

ACKNOWLEDGEMENTS

Much enthusiasm and support has helped me see this book through from concept to birth, and my special thanks go to all my students who have been so wonderfully responsive, to my parents, who have never tired of listening, my editor, Mary Banks, whose enthusiasm never flagged, Frances Denholm who typed away furiously at the manuscript, the models Penny Marlton, Mona Nachi, Kara Wales, Joan and Philip Winter, and my dear husband Peter, who has been a tower of strength to me throughout.

1984   **Jacki Winter**

The publishers are grateful to the following: Dr Stephen Greene of the John Radcliffe Hospital, Oxford for reading and commenting on the manuscript; Dr Rowan Hillson of the Radcliffe Infirmary, Oxford for permission to reproduce her photograph (page 31) of young diabetics at the Outward Bound Mountain School, Eskdale, Cumbria; Derek and Julia Parker for permission to reproduce the table on page 18 from *Do It Yourself Health* (Thames and Hudson); Adidas (Umbro International Footwear Ltd), Stockport, Cheshire, for loaning the shoes; Nike International Ltd, Washington, Tyne and Wear, and Pineapple Dance Studios, London for loaning the clothes; and the Reject Shop, London for the other props.

Photography was by Steve Powell/Allsport. The drawings are by David Gifford.

INDEX

Page numbers in *italic* refer to the illustrations.

Other books in the Positive Health Guide series

DIABETES
Dr James Anderson
A complete new guide to healthy living for diabetics,
featuring the recently developed high carbohydrate
and fibre (HCF) diet programme.

THE DIABETICS' DIET BOOK
Dr Jim Mann and the Oxford Dietetic Group
The first book for diabetics and their dietitians that
shows how to change to the new high carbohydrate
and fibre diet now recommended by leading diabetic
organizations.

THE DIABETICS' COOKBOOK
Roberta Longstaff, SRD and Dr Jim Mann
Following the international success of the bestselling
Diabetics' Diet Book, this sequel volume includes
special sections on cooking for children and food for
festive occasions.

Positive Health Programs for the Sinclair ZX
Spectrum 48K computer
(available only from Martin Dunitz Ltd, London)

DIABETES
Dr Peter Wise and Susan Farrant
Entertaining, interactive programs that tell you all you
need to know to control your condition, whether or not
you need insulin.

THE DIABETICS' DIET PROGRAM
Dr Tom Sanders
Personalized daily diet planning at the touch of a
button.